Lazarus: From Seven to Seventy-Seven

Lazarus: From Seven to Seventy-Seven

Eugene Weisberger

iUniverse, Inc.
New York Lincoln Shanghai

Lazarus: From Seven to Seventy-Seven

iUniverse, Inc.

For information address:
iUniverse, Inc.
2021 Pine Lake Road, Suite 100
Lincoln, NE 68512
www.iuniverse.com

ISBN: 0-595-31560-7

Printed in the United States of America

This autobiography is dedicated to my mother and father, Sabina Sprung Weisberger and Jacob Weisberger, who spent too few years with me, nevertheless will always be in my heart.

And to Lila Lizabeth my life-long companion and love. Both books, <u>The Chinese Walking Stick</u> and <u>Lazarus</u>, and all my stories are written with her sage advice and psychological understanding. Despite her very busy life in Poetry Therapy, she finds time to help me with many ideas, which make the volumes worthy. Her love and understanding have made our thirty-five years together just wonderful. My love for my wife is beyond words. She has been by my side in the good times and the difficult years.

And finally to all the children and grandchildren, whom I am sure will one day want to know the history and tales of their father and grandfather, I leave this book. Basically, it is for this reason I have taken to the computer in the first place.

In Memoriam:
My Two Mentors

Two men played a very important part in my management career, who showed me by their example the way toward management with integrity. During my early management years Ralph Mendel set a wonderful example of being a straight-shooter and treating all employees with understanding and kindness. He proved that one did not have to be a bully to gain respect with one's employees.

My feelings about him are best summarized in the following quote, which is one of my favorites:

There is nothing as strong as gentleness
or as gentle as real strength

Ralph Mendel was my boss and mentor for over ten years during the time I was formulating my management skills and philosophies about how important it was to treat people with care and dignity.

In my senior management years I was fortunate enough to take a two-year Advanced Management Training Seminar with Walter Mahler, who was a manager of unusual sorts. He did not spend time *in* industry, but rather *with* industry. He started a program that helped hundreds of the best executives in some of the largest companies in the country move up the ladder of success. Leadership to Walter was an art. He showed us how to enjoy it and participate in it. He made us understand that management meant excitement with teamwork. It was possible to make management fun by working with our fellow executives in constructive ways, making the business pay off, staying on top of your subject and working as a team to succeed.

I miss the sage advice of these two men who recently left us.

Contents

Acknowledgements

To all my FRIENDS and COWORKERS: As I look back at two generations of an exciting career, I realize how important all these people were to me both to succeed and to survive.

Whether it was meeting Ron Myer in Athens, or the Royal Air Force customer, Jim Brown in Sidney, Australia, or Georges DeCock in Au Provence, France; wherever I had contact with any of my associates there was a warmth, a sharing, a true companionship, no matter how many years after our relationship had ended.

During my working years there was always one man who was with me every step up the ladder of success, and someone I credit for making my career so much fun. Not only were we great work associates, but I can say that we were good friends as well. For my entire management role at General Instrument, Jim Adams was by my side with sound advice that was provided generously. My entire career would not have been the same without Jim.

I believe in one way or another all those people somehow or other helped me to survive. No matter how near or far, my friends have been so helpful during the difficult times. For example, there was Joel and Barbara Morris, who came to the hospital many times when I was relearning to walk. They stayed to talk with me as I recovered from one surgery after another, and were so helpful in getting me back to normality.

Another pair of friends who stood by Lila and me during the last ten years is Marty and Barbara Goodstone. Marty who traveled with me for about five years, and Barbara who was so available to support us in whatever way we needed. Finally there is my friend and cousin, Joe Burros, who traveled with me and stayed by my side through thick and thin.

Finally, I would like to acknowledge a special life-long relationship between Allan Mirkin and myself. We have been friends and pals for over seventy years. We shared many life experiences together beginning in first grade in P.S. 114 in Queens.

Allan Mirkin and I started out in the Boy Scouts in Troop 112; we were even in the same patrol, The Pine Tree. We were in the Navy at the same time, and met on numerous occasions in Chicago for fun and merrymaking.

When we were discharged after college, Allan became Scout Master of our old troop, and I became his assistant. Before he opened his optical practice, we would meet for lunch since we were friends, but also worked in the allied technical fields. We became telephone speaking buddies for a time while we both raised our families. In recent years, we have once again become good friends as we were in the beginning. I think it was basically because we liked each other.

In thinking back over the last few years, Allan and I shared important occasions with each other and our wives. For example, Lila and I attended Allan and Jean's 50th Wedding Anniversary. Later, Allan and Jean were at the book celebration that Lila gave for my first book The Chinese Walking Stick. I believe that sharing each other's moments of enjoyment help to cement a relationship.

What I remember most about Allan in the early years is a particular idiosyncrasy that he may not even want me to tell. During our elementary school days when we would line up to get injections for small pox or some such disease, I always stood behind him because I knew he was squeamish about getting shots, and I wanted to be there in case he fainted. I thought that's what friends were for.

After this book was almost complete, I realized the book required a professional review to take the ideas, thoughts, and tales into a more coherent, readable volume. I was fortunate to locate a person who was able to give Lazarus the polishing it needed. Although I have great ideas for short stories, I do not have the literary accomplishment necessary to make the book memorable. Johanna Martinez, a social worker and poetry expert brought the book a special understanding of literature and grammar to smooth out its rough edges over many hours.

I would like to especially acknowledge her great help in putting Lazarus into a finished product. After my 77th birthday, just as the book was being concluded, I had another bout of spinal problems. Lila and I rushed off to Sloan Kettering Hospital in Manhattan, and left Johanna to do much of this book's final review by herself. I am especially grateful for her last minute review. As soon as you read the stories you will agree with my choice of Johanna as editor and proofreader, par excellence.

Likewise, on the physical side, I am so thankful for Dr. Nessa Coyle who has helped me sort my medical issues over many years, and to Dr. Mark Bilsky for his continued concern and rapid response in fixing my back again.

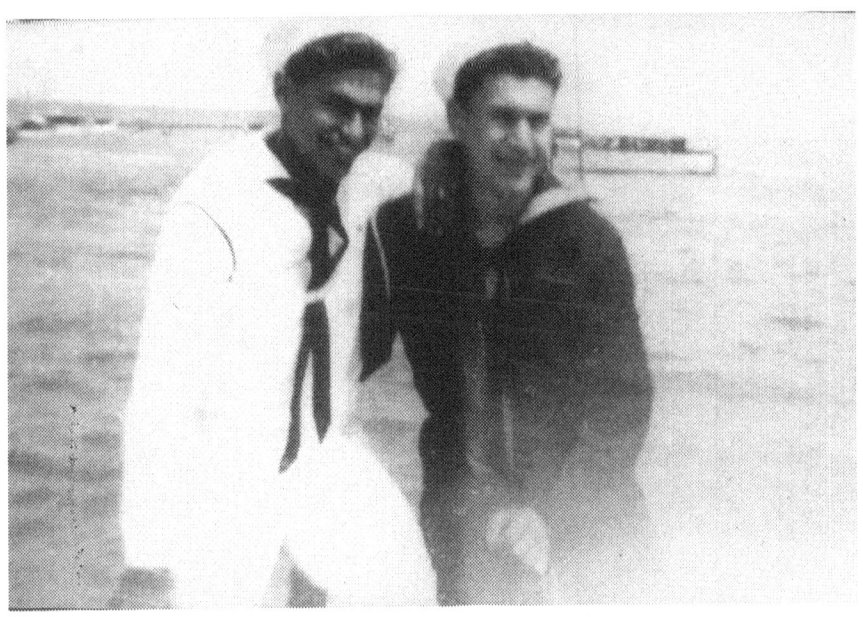

Gene and Allan Mirkin on the Navy Pier Chicago, Summer '45

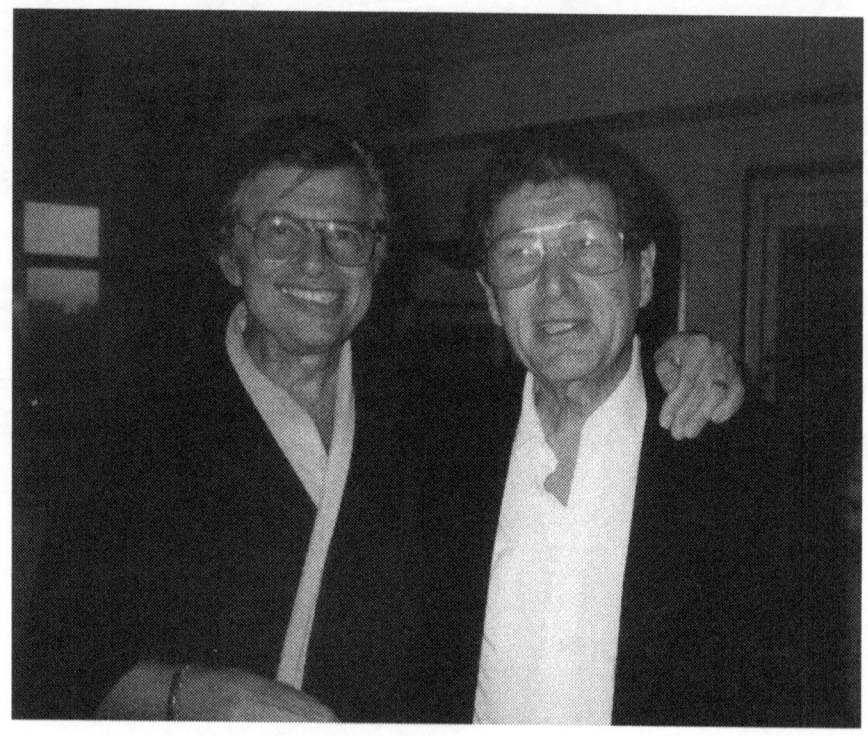

Gene and Allan Fifty-Five Years Later

Preface

Lazarus is a book of my life, my philosophies and my ideals. I have always felt that caring about people, for people and understanding people, makes for a good executive, a good husband and a family man. My ideals come from an environment and upbringing surrounded by strong family ties.

The stories in Lazarus come from my life's experiences as I have remembered them. From my earliest days I worked hard, selflessly and at the same time enjoying what I did. I learned the value and importance of success, but not at the price of stepping over others.

I learned that in order to be successful one needs a well-rounded education. My years at Brooklyn Tech High School, Brooklyn Poly and NYU Graduate School all came in very handy in the formulation of my working career.

Lastly, I learned that one needed a positive attitude about life and, as Poet Laureate Stanley Kunitz said, "Live in the layers, not on the litter." For me those layers involved many levels of professional experience, many interactions with lots of people in all parts of the business world, and it also brought me in contact with people from all over the world that was both exciting and rewarding. I had the good fortune to work with wonderful people in an exciting career and in the process visit so many different places around the world. My first book, The Chinese Walking Stick, described my travels around the world before and after my illness.

Lazarus tells of my life in an introspective way from my earliest days until the present. I have been blessed with an excellent memory and now in my later years I have been able to recall many experiences and incidents from almost seventy years. In the past seven years I wrote many stories on the Internet, but I realized that assembling a volume is far more inclusive and permits the reader to get a much better view of a total scene.

Chapters One through Four are the chronological presentation of seventy years of my life. Chapter Five presents a view of a fun part of life, which has helped me overcome many difficult times. It is having fun with kids, which has helped me to get over hard times.

Chapter Six includes stories I just loved to write and you may find fun to read. They are not chronological nor travel but they are experiences from my "reservoir of life's layers."

Finally, the book concludes with a final chapter of more remembrances and surprises from life, which were great fun, as well as a last look at the philosophy of life as I see it.

Introduction

Lazarus: From Seven To Seventy-Seven

Now that <u>The Chinese Walking Stick</u> is complete and in publication, I can think of the book I did not write. Although <u>The Chinese Walking Stick</u> is basically a travel book, it also includes several stories about travel under difficult conditions. In a wheelchair or with a cane, I just kept on going.

<u>Lazarus: From Seven to Seventy-seven</u> is a collection of my memoirs. The book omits certain sensitive parts of my life whose inclusion may cause some discomfort to some family members. The one great aspect of an autobiography is that the author includes what he wishes and omits what he chooses.

This new book, <u>Lazarus</u>, deals to a much greater extent with my struggles with pain and life in general. How my background of almost seventy years of battling and determination prepared me for the fight of my life. I did not know it at the time but each incident was a preparation for that war.

The story in the New Testament talks about Jesus bringing back Lazarus from the dead. One would ask why a Jew would pick the name Lazarus for his autobiography. The name really has nothing to do with religion, but with the concept of living on the brink and coming back with good fortune. I was named Lazarus by one of my oncologists, Dr. David Pfister since I kept bouncing back after illness.

The story begins with my earliest recollections of the traumatic time of my mother's accident as it coincided with my father's untimely death. From the first day when my mother came home from the hospital and told me that," now I would be the man of the family," the battle began. Then going to school to face the embarrassment of the students to feel that they knew I no longer had a father. I felt as though I was known, during my entire elementary education as "the boy without a father." Chapter One continues with my tales of growing up in the depression. I grew up with lots of excitement and hard work, like most boys in the Depression.

In Chapter Two when I joined the Navy World War II was almost over, and I never thought I was in danger, but surprisingly a train crash outside of Cincinnati could have ended my life all too prematurely. A fortuitously relocation of four empty railroad cars saved the two hundred men of our company from getting wiped out. In the service I never left the country, but my bout with pneumonia could have had disastrous consequences. I have often thought about my grandmother and grandfather (my Mother's Mother and Father) deaths due to pneumonia, and probably would have survived if penicillin had been discovered a generation or two earlier. Conversely, I was saved by Pfizer's development of penicillin and was in the right place at the right time. Then in a way, getting pneumonia prevented me from becoming a radio-gunner, which could very well have put me in harm's way during the last very dangerous months of the war.

My career was full of excitement and Chapter Three tells many stories of my promotions and of the division's successes. I think you will find them interesting, fun and worth reading. My first book, described many of my travels, but not very much about the business aspect of my life. Here in Chapter Three you will get a feeling of my management style.

Over the course of twenty years, I moved up slowly but surely at Radio Receptor/General Instrument. I was not like a shooting star, but moved with determination and morality of example. If I had to describe myself, I would be more like the tortoise, and not the hare. I moved up each step of the way with care and understanding of the workers who stayed with me on the trip. Those personality traits also helped me overcome my disease. I never gave up, always fought to the bitter end, but at the same I tried to concern myself with the other person.

During my early years with the company I had a minor operation that was so trivial it hardly rated a story. A small benign growth was removed from my neck while I was in my mid-twenties. For forty or more years as I worked my way up the business ladder the remnants of that tiny tumor slowly and insidiously were doing its damage. During those two generations, I never gave the slightest thought to what was happening inside my neck.

After I retired, I continued traveling, which helped motivate me to share my tales with my many readers. In 1996 Lila and I made plans to visit the last of the continents—Antarctica, but alas "the best laid plans of mice and travelers..." As we were ready to leave I was hit with the most dreaded of diseases and have spent the last eight years battling cancer. In Chapter Four I write about my struggle with illness and pain. It is a battle that even now I must continue fighting.

After I was hit with cancer, I wanted to tell the stories from my life of work, fun and excitement. I was fortunate to be quite healthy during my four decades with General Instrument and discovered that remembering the good times and writing stories is an important part of my healing. I found I had interesting tales to tell that have stuck with me for scores of years, and writing was such a great way to express oneself. Almost two hundred stories found in The Chinese Walking Stick and Lazarus were written without referring to a single recorded note.

After the intensity of Chapter Four: The Illness, the book takes a turn to the lighter side. I realize that humor and fun are so important to survival. I have included the Kiddie stories of Chapter Five to remind me that in the midst of the tension, there is also laughter and fun, and it often involves children. I have been fortunate enough to live with some of my grandchildren for the last few years, and having them by my side has helped me forget my troubles. When Rachel and Matthew climb into my bed and we turn the television on to watch everything from the World News to "Sponge Bob" and "Hey, Arnold!" I can feel my tension ease away. There are many varieties of "tension relievers." There is tai chi, dance and poetry therapy, even "puppy dog therapy." For me, "Sponge Bob Therapy" with Matthew and Rachel is one of the best.

But the world is full of trials and tribulations of all sorts and extremes. Chapter Six puts some of these into perspective. These five short stories cover a span of over hundred years and a variety of subjects, personal to worldly, from light to darkness, from beautiful to horrendous from moral to immoral. It is a mixture of tales of the nineteenth and twentieth centuries.

Finally, in Chapter Seven, I go back to personal tales of special celebrations of my life. I once again remember life can be fun, especially with loving and caring family and friends.

Now, to my tales.

Chapter One: Growing Up

Dedicated to my mother and father: Sabina and Jacob

1. NOW YOU ARE THE MAN OF THE FAMILY

The winter of '34 was a particularly vicious one because there was one snowstorm after another. My mother was a spunky little gray haired lady who had just turned forty-six, but never thought to dye her hair. In spite of the harsh winter, one day she decided to take my sister, Rita and I to visit my father's relatives in Brooklyn. It was a sad time for the family because my father's oldest brother, Uncle Sam, had just died from cancer and in the Jewish tradition we went to pay a shiva call.

In February the days are dark in New York and by five o'clock in the afternoon, a bleak and dark night sets in. We left Aunt Hannah's somber house on 19th Street in Brooklyn and took the bus for the rather long trip to Belle Harbor. At that time I was seven years old and Rita was nine years old, and I always remember my mother as looking rather elderly for a lady with young children. My mother had a sweet smile and a happy disposition. As I look back at her life I am sure that I have many of her traits. She always looked at the sunny side of things in life, as I do.

This February evening we stood huddled in the cold night air while waiting to board the ferry on the Brooklyn side of Jamaica Bay. In those days there was no Marine Park Bridge to span the Bay. The ferry was the only way to get from Brooklyn to Rockaway's Belle Harbor. I remember the boat was rather small, with a twenty-car capacity, and a closed-in room with a heated stove where about thirty or so walk-on passengers would sit on the wooden benches for the twenty-minute ride to the Rockaway. The ferry left Brooklyn and pulled up to its slip in Rockaway without incident. We were the last to disembark from the ferry, and walked slowly off the boat and along the passenger walkway.

The Rockaway Beach Boulevard bus did not go right to the ferry, but made its final stop about 100 yards from the boat slip.

The three of us walked carefully from the boat to the bus stop. Because the ground was icy, my mother held my sister and me in each hand.

All of a sudden our whole life changed. My mother slipped and fell to the icy ground. We could see that she was unable to get up, and that she was in severe pain. She just lay there motionless, and Rita and I also stood there paralyzed with fear. It was obvious that she was badly hurt and what was equally bad was that there was no one to help.

My sister and I just stood there petrified. We were quite a distance from the bus stop, but close to the entrance of the U.S. Army Base at Fort Tilden. After several minutes a car driven by a soldier pulled up to the gate and stopped. He got out and asked if we needed help. My mother said that she could not move and asked that he please take us to our home in Belle Harbor.

The soldier drove us to my grandmother's house on Beach 130th Street. He went to the door and rang the bell. In a minute my father came down the long flight of steps, and carried my mother up two flights to her bedroom.

Minutes later I could hear the siren of the ambulance coming down our street. By then I was in my room, but could hear the commotion all over the house. The next thing I knew, the ambulance screeched its way up the block, taking my mother to Rockaway Beach Hospital.

The next few days were a living nightmare. Either the maid or our grandma would give us meals, but I remember very little else. My grandmother told us my mother had a broken leg, but later on I found out that it was far worse than I had been informed and it was broken in three places.

For days I watched my father and uncles pace around the house, but they hardly talked to my sister or me. Then a day or two later, I saw my father in his woolen bathrobe, walking solemnly around the house. The following morning two uncles told me my father had been taken to the same hospital as my mother, and *he* was going have an operation the next day.

I was in a complete state of confusion, and just too little to know what was going on, while family members walking all over the house. Shock and fear gripped me. Nobody told me what was going on but I knew whatever was going on, was very bad. Everyone was whispering to each other, and they would stop talking as soon as I entered the room. Days went by and I went from fear into panic. Still no one talked to me. I remember that as soon as the telephone would ring some family member would answer it, take it to the basement stairs, closing the door, so I could not hear.

Then one day I remember the entire house go from crowded with relatives to a state of complete emptiness. I roamed around that big house in utter dismay.

Just what was going on I did not know. Later on in life, I discovered that this was the day of my father's funeral.

The maid stayed at home with my sister and me, while my mother lay in the hospital with her broken leg, and the rest of the family attended my father's funeral. Members of the family did not know how to tell us about our father, so they decided to wait for my mother to return. We just walked around day after day in a stupor.

After what seemed to be weeks, an ambulance drove up to the front of the house and my mother was carried on a stretcher to her second floor bedroom of the big house. The maid called Rita, and me and said that Mama wanted to see us.

As we walked down from the third floor to Mama's room on the second floor, it seemed to be the longest minute of my young life. We each sat at the foot of the bed. My mother was propped up with pillows all around her. Her cast looked like a huge canopy covering her leg from hip to toes. She put a hand out to each of us and said, "I have such bad news. Papa died last week." All three of us just cried and cried.

Then Mama looked at me and said. "Eugene, you are now the man of the family."

I could not say a word. Nothing but tears flowed from my eyes. I just squeezed Mama's hand and I thought, now I would have to be am a man!

It is now seventy years later and I cannot think of that moment without getting tears in my eyes.

2. BACK TO P.S. 114

Springtime finally arrived in my sad town of Belle Harbor and I had to think about going back to school after my father's passing. My mom was still in a cast and I was quite reluctant to face the world after my father's death. One day at the end of March, my Uncle Sol, one of three uncles who still lived with Grandma in our big house on 130th street, took me by the hand and said I had to go back to school this week.

I found all three of my bachelor uncles that lived with us to be very considerate and nice. Uncle Sol was the oldest of the three, kind and gentle, Uncle Percy was next, intellectual and somewhat distant, and Uncle Dave was always thought of as the baby of the family of twelve, and was the happy-go-lucky little man of the family. Percy and Dave would go to New York each day for their businesses, but Sol had the real estate office on 116th St. in Rockaway Beach. It was easy for him to take me to school because he set his own hours. I was always so proud of my family in Rockaway, but felt especially proud of the Sprung Bros. Realty Office in the very center of town.

But on the day I had to return to P.S. 114 I was not thinking of any of those highlights because I was more worried about facing the kids in my class. What would I say to them or what would they say to me? What would they think? The worst feeling I had was one of guilt. I almost felt responsible for all this.

I was both embarrassed and scared. I thought all my friends would look at me, and I would not know what to say. On the way to school, Uncle Sol held me by the hand, but did not say much either. I do not think anyone said anything that day.

We went up to the teacher's desk and Uncle Sol started talking to her. The only thing that I heard him tell the teacher was that my father was deceased. Since I had never heard that word before, my little mind thought that it was possible that this word had a more positive meaning. Perhaps my mother was wrong and that maybe Daddy was in a hospital somewhere, and that deceased meant that he would be coming back soon. But this was not the case, so I walked slowly to my seat with my head down. I cannot remember a single thing that anyone said that day.

Sadly, when I saw Uncle Dave that night, I cautiously asked Him, "What does deceased mean?" Uncle Dave's eyes opened wide, and I could see the tears roll down his cheeks. I went to sit on his lap, while he sat quietly for a long time. Then for the second time, I heard that my father had died.

3. A Secret Revealed

For four months from September to December 1939, I rode my bike to Temple Beth El for Bar Mitzvah lessons. I had a nice young teacher, Mr. Douglas, instructing me; that is until the very last week. Then Dr. Robert Gordus, Rabbi of Temple Beth El, took over the final instruction. He was a tall serious man with dark black hair and a deep voice. He had the kind of voice that would scare little kids who were not accustomed to it. Every Friday evening and Saturday morning I would go the Temple to see other boys of my class go through the ritual.

Finally, it was going to be my turn. I was scheduled for a dress rehearsal on the Thursday night before the Saturday of my Bar Mitzvah. This meant that you would stand up at the lectern and go through your entire Haftorah (the part of the ritual assigned to you). Rabbi Gordus in his long black robe, and his little black yarmulke, said, "All right, Eugene, begin." As I started, he left the podium and walked to the rear of the sanctuary. He went behind the last row and walked back and forth with his hands clasped behind his back. As I began reading, I suddenly heard his booming voice say, "Louder!" I increased the volume of my changing voice the best way I could. In another few seconds, as he paced back and forth, came another, "Louder!" Obviously he was showing me by example what he meant by louder, as his booming voice resonated all over the Temple. There was no way that my young voice could possibly compete with his. I felt totally inadequate, but I did the best I could, as he would continue his instructive single word "Louder."

At last I finished my rehearsal performance thinking that Saturday would surely be a disaster. On Friday evening my family and I went to temple and I had to give the prayer over the wine. That worked out all right, but the next day was the real test. Would I be able to rise to the occasion? I knew I just could not raise my voice as loud as Rabbi Gordus wanted me to. I was convinced that it was going to be a mess. Was there anything that could get me out of this predicament? Yes, there was.

Friday night the temple burned down. I was free and would not have to put on my performance. Oh what a relief!

But lo and behold! I woke up Saturday morning to my mother's usual, "Rise and shine!" But this time she added, "Today is your big day."

"Oh damn it, I must have dreamt it. The temple must still be there."

At nine o'clock we walked to Beach 122nd Street to see the temple still standing. Minutes later I would hear Dr. Gordus call me to the podium to say my Haftorah. Somehow or other my voice was clear as a bell and louder than ever.

Everyone said I did well. At last it was over, and I never told anyone how I dreamt the temple burned down.

4. MY FIRST JOBS

In 1938 I was eleven years old. My father had been gone for about five years. Grandma had been gone for almost two years. Her big house had been sold and the money was divided among her twelve children. We were still in the heart of the Depression. The number of unemployed mentioned at the dinner table was sixteen million Americans. My mother did not have a job, but stayed at home trying to make ends meet.

My mother, sister, and I were living on Beach 127th Street in Belle Harbor, in a five room apartment, one block from the Atlantic Ocean. The highlight of my existence was living one hundred yards from the Atlantic Ocean. I loved walking on the beach all year long, especially in the spring and fall, also known as the period before and after the summer crowds came to the beaches.

The summers had one special treat for me during my early years. It was watching the fireworks fired off a barge in the ocean after dark. Every Wednesday evening at nine o'clock many of my friends would come out on the warm summers nights and walk along the boardwalk to watch the beautiful display. Although fireworks have become a lot more spectacular in the past sixty years, it made no difference to us since we did not know any better in the 1930's and thought they were the greatest. No matter what the problems were with money or paying the rent, when Wednesday night rolled around, all would melt in the brilliant flashes that streaked across the sky. The boardwalk was jammed with all of the town's people, who watched in awe and let out the "Ah" sound I became so familiar with.

I loved to walk to the amusement center on 116th Street and watch the men play pinball machines, and compete in rolling balls into holes on a table. There must have been fifty tables and people sat at them all night long at a nickel a game. Getting five in a row first would get you a prize ticket. My Uncle Dave was an expert player, so I always felt so proud when his bell rang and the owner came over to give him a ticket. All summer long my uncle would save up his winning tickets to use at the end of the season and buy us some prizes.

But it was Thursday morning and reality came too soon. Before we knew it the rent was due again. Our biggest expense was the monthly rent. Because our income was low we shared the apartment with some of my uncles to reduce our expenses. One big source of income for our family was to rent out three of our five rooms during the summer months to families from New York City who wanted to get away from the city's heat. In the 1930's air conditioning was only a thought for the future.

We rented out two bedrooms and the kitchen, and moved our kitchen down into the basement. Back then we only had an icebox and would get a big piece of ice every few days. Of course, the ice would melt and the water would run down into the pan under the box. My job was to empty the pan every day. It was not a hard job, so long as I remembered to do it. Every once in a while, I would forget, and the basement kitchen would get soaked. My memory was tickled when I walked into the kitchen and saw water flooding the floor. My mother would not yell or get angry. She would simply say, "Mop up the floor."

One summer we had a family whose father was a semi-professional baseball player with the New York Giants. It was my only interaction with a real live ballplayer, and I loved to hear him talk about baseball. One afternoon he actually took us to a ball game. His son and three of us from the block went to the Polo Grounds to watch the Giants play. It was an exciting game although the Giants lost, but for the next sixty years I remained a Giants fan.

In the winter, my job was to shovel out the furnace ashes in the morning, and put in the new coals for the day. If I ever forgot, the house would suddenly become ice cold. In this situation, I would race down to the basement to see the last of the flicker coals go out, and then I would restart the coal stove. This required paper, sticks, matches, and anything else available to get it started again. It was one big pain in the neck, so I did not forget too often.

Because the jobs inside the house did not get me any pocket money, I decided one day I had to go out and earn some cash. Two blocks from our house on Beach 129th Street, was an entire block of little stores. I started at the corner nearest Newport Avenue, and methodically when into every store to ask if they needed any one to help. No one was hiring anybody in those days, so by the time I reached the end of the long street with twenty or so stores, I was pretty discouraged.

I tried all the grocery stories, vegetable markets and the candy stories, even the beauty parlor! (Not that I knew what I could do in a beauty parlor.)

The last store on the street was a butcher shop, called Steingart's Meat Market. When I asked Nat Steingart if he needed any help, he said that he had a delivery boy. But, he thought it over for a minute and then with hesitation said, "The boy I have has not been working out too well. Let me think it over. Give me your phone number and I will call you if I can use you." Two days later, I received a call from Nat.

"Can you start tomorrow afternoon?" he said.

I said, "Sure, what time?"

He said, "From three to six."

I was so thrilled that I forgot to ask how much he would pay. However I reported to work at five minutes to three the next day. My job was to deliver packages of meat all over Belle Harbor, Rockaway Beach and Neponsit. When I had Neponsit deliveries I considered it as both good and bad news. Neponsit began at 142nd Street so it was a long trip on my bicycle. On the other hand, the ladies in Neponsit were usually rich and tipped the most. I often got a dime, which I thought was just outrageous.

At the end of the week, I received my pay envelope with three dollars for the twelve hours I had worked. My salary was a great big twenty-five cents an hour, but it felt so good to have three dollars in my pocket. Also, the tips were enough for my milk money, so I did not have to ask my mother for it.

After working for a short time Mr. Steingart said I would have to get a Social Security card. I had heard about Social Security in school, but now I actually had an opportunity to experience it. It was the first transaction I ever had with the government. I filled out the form and had Mr. Steingart sign it, and to this day, my card has his name on it.

I worked there for almost two years without ever missing a day. Although delivering packages was sometimes very tedious, especially when there was snow on the ground, I was the kind of person who stuck to what I had to do, come hell or high water. This personality trait has been a part of my life and I believe has helped me to succeed. I never knew it, but it must have been in my genes.

5. TODAY I AM A LAWN MOWER

The most majestic of signs stands on the corner of 34th Street and Broadway and reads, "Macy's The World's Largest Department Store." I never understood how they measured this declaration, but I also never met anyone who disputed this fact. Macy's is so big that it covers one entire city block from Broadway to Seventh Ave and 34th Street to 35th Street, and is twelve stores high. The year I went to apply for a job the employment office was on the mezzanine floor. I sat in a large auditorium with hundreds of young men and women applying for Christmas jobs in 1946. Christmas was the biggest shopping season of the year; therefore Macy's hired hundreds of young people to meet the holiday rush. My application indicated that I had lots of experience: a delivery boy at a butcher shop, a stockman at the five and dime and most importantly a U. S. Navy veteran.

The interview lasted about five minutes, but on the bottom of the application was the all-important: *Hired. Begin 12/4/46. $0.90/hr.* In those days ninety cents an hour seemed like a fortune.

I arrived the next Saturday morning bright and early at the employment office to be given an assignment. Dozens of department heads and others wore red or white carnations, ready to pick out their "tempos" for the season. A tall, dark man came up to me and asked my name. His badge said, *Dietz, Gardening.*

"Where do you live?" he asked.

I said, "In Flatbush, Brooklyn, sir."

"In a private house or apartment?" He asked further.

"Apartment House," I said, "On Ocean Avenue, 1866." I volunteered further, thinking he wanted my address. I did not understand the exact reason for all of these questions because my address was on the application he was holding.

He looked rather disappointed, but said, "OK! Come with me."

He wore a dark suit and had a red carnation in his lapel, which I assumed meant he was a big shot. We took the elevator down to the basement and I followed him to the back of the store, which was not opened to customers yet. Looking around the store, I noticed people were busy doing things that I knew nothing about. Mr. Dietz seemed to stop by everyone to give instructions, answer questions or move signs around, and on and on. All of a sudden he must have remembered that I was tagging along behind him. He turned around and said words I would remember for a long time, "You are in lawn mowers." That was a complete shock. My knowledge of lawn mowers could be written on a blade of grass.

There it was nine o'clock in the morning at Macy's when suddenly the bells went off, and the doors opened. People came racing in like "The Charge of the Light Brigade." Over the years I became accustomed to those Saturday crowds before Christmas, but that first Saturday was a day to remember.

People raced in with circulars or newspapers under their arms trying to get the holiday sales. Often there was only a limited amount of each type of item available at the sale prices, so people tried to get it before it sold out. Shoppers would race up to you and ask, "Where is this or where is that?" I was in a complete daze. I stood next to my beloved lawn mowers hoping nobody would dare ask me a question about them. I touched each one lovingly and tried to look as though I knew what they were all about.

In those days the mowers were all manual, except the rotary models which were electric. On the first day an elderly woman asked me which of the mowers was easiest to push. Now I did not have the slightest idea which one to recommend. But I hesitated, as if I was thinking it over.

She pressed further, "Which one do you use?"

I did not have the nerve to say, "We do not use lawn mowers in our three room fourth floor apartment in Flatbush."

Instead, I said, "I think this one is the best." I pointed to the most expensive one. Fortunately, she said, "I will think it over."

Over the next four Thursday nights and Saturdays, I gradually became more knowledgeable about those machines. After the Christmas season ended, January came around and hundreds of tempos found themselves out of work again. We were expected to work until the end of the calendar year to help with returns, which over the years I thought was a bigger business than the pre-holiday sales. During the last week of December, I was given my schedule for January and was informed that I was not longer a "tempo" and would be working part time from then on. I guess I learned more about lawn mowers than I thought. When power mowers arrived, I actually knew what a "horsepower" was.

I stayed at Macy's for four years and learned about every nut and bolt of each lawn mower in the store; eventually becoming the store's expert. Over the years, I often told my friends about selling lawn mowers while living in an apartment house. When they laughed, I would say, "Look, you don't have to be a chicken to know how to make a good chicken soup."

6. THE MACY TWINS: HARRIET & JACKIE

Saturdays were always exhausting days at Macy's. No matter how many years I worked there, I was always tired because standing on my feet was such a strain. By the time I worked for three hours or so all I Could think about was sitting down. Lunch was usually at 12:00 and I would go up to the cafeteria, get a sandwich and rest. One day I saw a rather nice looking brunette sitting alone and reading. I often did not have enough nerve to join anyone, but somehow that day I decided to be a bit aggressive and sat down at her table.

"What are you reading?" I asked. She answered with a smile and in time we were deep in conversation. She introduced herself as Harriet and told me she was going to Brooklyn College for education. She worked in the shoe department and had also been lucky enough to be tapped for a permanent job after Christmas. Before long, my lunch-hour was over. I said something like I hoped to see her next week, but was not confident enough to ask for her phone number. Going to an all boys college did not give me much of an opportunity to meet girls. Meanwhile, the gardening department consisted of Mr. Dietz and about one half dozen middle-aged women. Harriet was the first contact I made since joining Macy's and it felt really great. That Saturday afternoon just flew by. I thought about meeting Harriet the following week and imagined all the things I would talk about to overcome my shyness. Where did she live? What year was she in college? And lots of other questions came to mind. With an afternoon spent daydreaming, the six o'clock bell came quickly and then I headed for the subway.

The going home routine began with a race to the Broadway and 34th Street subway stop, charging down two flights of steps, putting my nickel in the slot and darting for the BMT Coney Island train. The trains and platforms were jammed with people all heading in the same direction. Most of the time I did not get a seat, but every once in a while I was lucky enough to see an empty one. Because the trains were coming from uptown, they were typically pretty crowded by the time they arrived at 34th Street. Usually I would have to stand until the Church Avenue station in Brooklyn when the trains would empty out enough to get a seat. That Saturday I remember getting a seat because it was so rare.

Just as I sat down and the train was about to depart, guess who rushed through the closing doors. It was Harriet from lunch. Boy! What a lucky break! But, there went my seat. I stood up and motioned to her to take it. I think she looked rather surprised, I suppose because in New York no one offers anyone a hard won subway seat.

She sat down with a smile and I started talking to her.

"What station do you get off at?" I asked.

But she seemed rather hesitant to talk. "Ah! Church Ave" she said.

"How's your book coming?" I asked.

"Okay." was her noncommittal answer. Clearly, she was not friendly like she was at lunch. I attributed this to the fact that she was tired. I stood near her for a while, but because she was not talking, my shyness took over, and I gradually moved away, feeling somewhat discouraged.

As usual the train got more and more crowded as we went further downtown toward the East River. Before I knew it we were in Brooklyn and a few minutes later Harriet got off at Church Ave. When she got off we smiled to each other and our meeting was at an end. I was very discouraged. All the questions I was going to ask at our next meeting never were said. My daydreams came to a frustrating end. But somehow or other my intense college curriculum did not leave me much time for sadness, so in a few days she was all but out of my mind.

That was until the following Saturday when I was heading up to the cafeteria and Harriet was on line in front of me.

"How was your week?" I asked.

"Great, she said with a smile."

"Do you want to sit here?" she asked.

"OK." I answered.

As we put our trays down she said, "Oh! There is my sister. Do you know Jackie?" I looked up and did a double take. There was another Harriet. I could not believe my eyes. There were two girls who looked absolutely identical.

Then Harriet said, "Jackie, this is Gene." I stared at them in complete disbelief. How could two people look so alike?

Jackie said with a slight smile, "I think you saw me on the subway last week." I was too flustered to say anything. So, that was whom I saw in the subway last week, I thought.

I was now certain that it must have been Jackie to whom I spoke with on the train going home. I looked back and forth at these two very pretty ladies and could not tell them apart. They both looked at me and laughed at my confusion. How could I tell them apart? When I thought about it, I concluded that Harriet had a happy smile, whereas Jackie was not nearly as friendly or so I thought. But sometimes when Harriet was tired, she wore a frown, and then again there were times when Jackie wore a smile. It was terribly confusing.

It did not help my dilemma that their job at Macy's was in the same shoe department. So I could not tell them apart by their department. I think they took a sadistic desire in confusing all their friends. They both went to Brooklyn

College; both wanted to become teachers; both lived at home with their parents. Every time I would figure out some trait or other to distinguish them, I would get thrown for a loop by mixing them up again.

I knew I wanted to become friendly with Harriet, but the only trouble was I did not know who Harriet was. I believe that most of the people who knew them just decided that it was too much trouble to try to separate them, so maybe it really did not make any difference. Of course, it did when you were trying to decide which one to date. It did not help that they also dressed identically and had the similar personality traits and characteristics.

I finally said that they were fun to be with, but it was just too much of an effort to get to know who was who. So we stayed Macy's friends and nothing more.

7. AT LAST: AN ENGINEER

The year 1950 was one of those bad years for graduating college. When President Rogers made his commencement address to the graduating class at Brooklyn Poly, he presented us with a very discouraging view regarding employment. He said that the number of engineering graduates was large, and the number of opportunities at that time was relatively small. His advice to us was very helpful in a way. He said the market will eventually expand and we should be patient. He concluded, "Take whatever job you can find, even if it is selling shoes at Thom McCann."

I left the auditorium in a glum mood. I could not believe that after spending almost four years working my tail off during the week, and working weekends at Macy's, that I would not be able to find a decent job. But those were the facts of the industrial life and I had to make the best of it. I applied at dozens of companies, but most of the time I could not even get an interview. I decided to stay at Macy's temporarily until something better came along.

In the meantime my Uncle Dave asked around at several electrical contractors to see if there were any openings. A small electrical contractor named Triangle Electric found temporary work for me in their shop repairing motors. The owner, Harvey Kramer, had about one-half dozen electricians installing motors and machines for the millinery trade.

As soon as I went to work there I found that he had no system for keeping track of his material costs as well as the time his workers spent on the job. Instead of repairing the damaged equipment, I was more useful by setting up a job cost system for his contracts that would bill his customers for the proper charges. In effect, I made my own job and Mr. Kramer did not seem to mind at all. He had no reason to mind because he was only paying me $40.00 a week and I was saving him many times that amount.

When I graduated college in June 1950 I applied for a job at the U. S. Navy Material Laboratory. About six months after starting at Triangle, a position became available at the Navy Material Lab. I took the job immediately since it was more than twice the salary than my Triangle position. The civil service position for graduate engineers, categorized as P-1, started at $5,200 a year plus vacation, sick leave and medical benefits. In those days it seemed like a million dollars. My friends and family could not believe that I would be earning $100 per week. I stayed at the Navy Yard for over a year testing equipment used on subs.

As I reflect on this particular job, I could have spent my entire career there living with the security of benefits and periodic pay increases. Many of the men in that department did exactly that, but that type of job was not exciting enough for me. I needed a challenging job, the kind of position that would fit with my inner drive.

Consequently, I woke up one day with the realization that civil service was not for me. I spoke to one of my uncles, who was a sales engineer, and told him I would like a more exciting job. Uncle Joe said he would inquire at some of the companies he represented.

A few weeks later he set up an interview for me. It was then that I realized the importance of contacts. There were at least six people applying for the job, but my uncle knew the president. I found out that day that one good word from the president is worth an entire paragraph from the personal assistant. The following week I resigned from the Navy Yard and started work at Radio Receptor as an engineer. I retired thirty-nine years later as Group President.

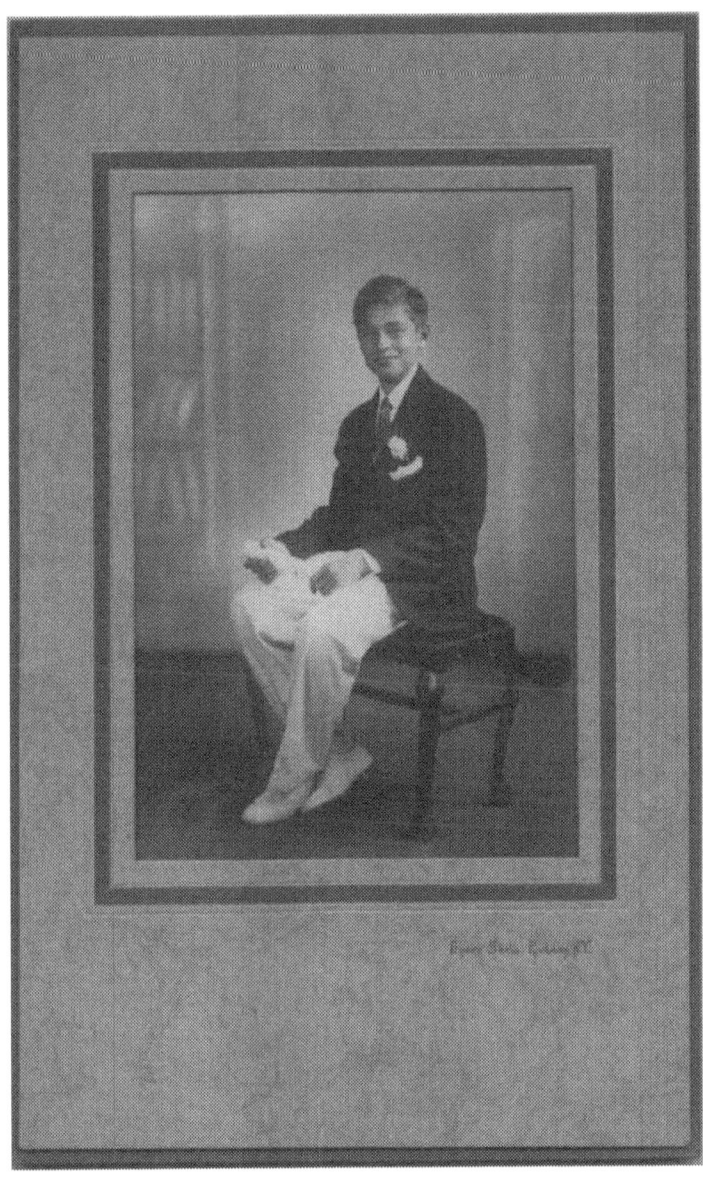

Gene at Thirteen, Belle Harbor, NY

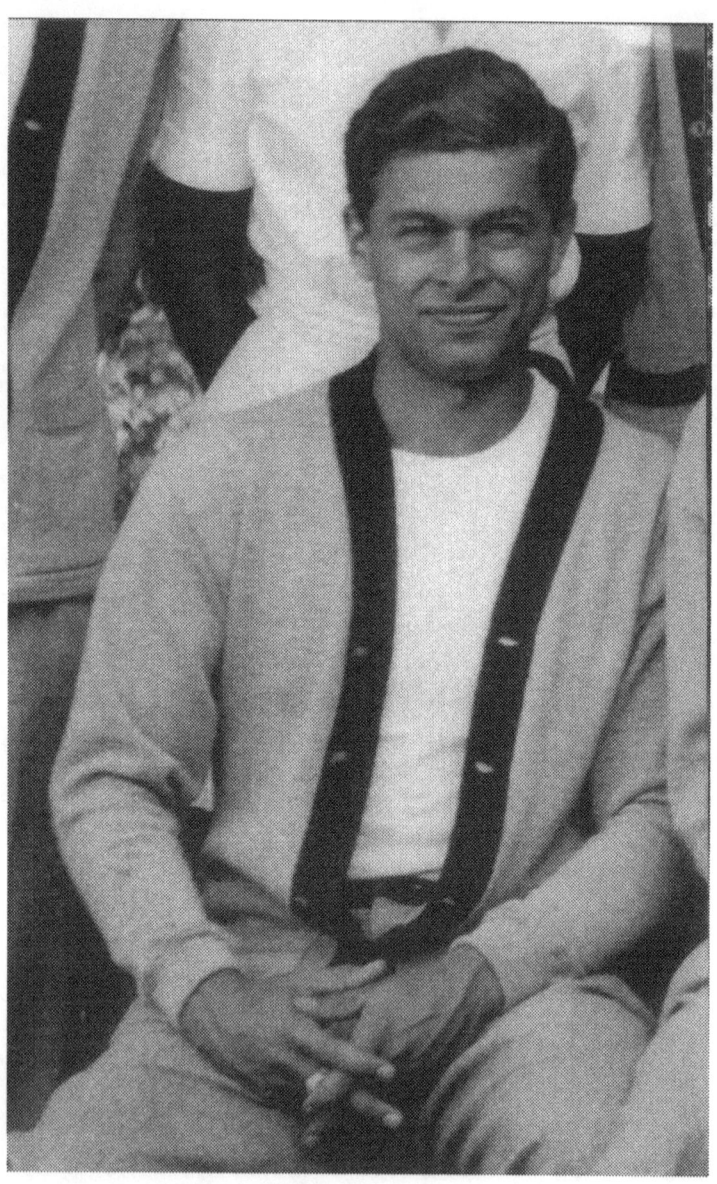

Gene at Camp Onota, Pittsfield, Mass.

Chapter Two: In Service

Dedicated to Cousin Donald Burros

1. THE TRAIN WRECK

Donald and I and left Penn station with about 200 others in the middle of November in 1944 because we had just enlisted in the Naval Air Force. Our plan was to go to school to either become pilots or technicians depending how we did in basic training school and our length of stay. The war was actively affecting every able bodied man to do something.

My cousin Donald had planned to join the Marine Corps, but my Aunt Flora convinced him to join the Navy after she learned that this was my plan. Donald's mother was certain that the Navy was safer. He was almost the last one to join the company before we left for basic training.

Two weeks before my 18th birthday I was scheduled to leave for the Naval Air Training Center in Memphis, Tennessee. Because I had completed my first semester at Brooklyn Poly, I would be able to continue my education when I got back. We were on our way to one of the largest Naval Centers in the East. We were told that we would train in Memphis for eight weeks, and then be assigned to one of three schools: pilot training, radio, or mechanical.

So, I said goodbye to all my family and friends in November 1944. The next morning I met with my cousin Donald at the train station. Traveling to Memphis by train from Brooklyn seemed to be very far away, but this was the age before regularly scheduled commercial airlines. It was a long train, and servicemen were seated in the first four cars, while the rest of the train was filled with business people.

We left about an hour later as the train moved out to the South and West. Most of the business people got off in Newark, New Jersey or Philadelphia, Pennsylvania. We rode down in cars that were especially designed for military use. Our car had four levels of sleeping bunks. We were scheduled to stay overnight on our one thousand mile journey that went by at an incredibly slow pace. The train lumbered its way through New Jersey, then Pennsylvania and finally moved into Ohio. It is difficult for me to describe to anyone in this century how long the trip from New York to Tennessee took in 1944.

By the time it was around eight at night, they brought in sandwiches for the second time in the day. Sometime during the trip, the railroad men put four additional empty cars between our cars and the locomotive. They told us that another few hundred Navy recruits would sit in those four additional cars. Little did we know that this simple action probably saved our lives. That night the train moved slowly through the outskirts of Cincinnati. We were all assigned to bunks, four decks high. I was in the second level, and my cousin, Donald, was in the bunk below me. We met several other Navy recruits from Boston and New Haven who were in the bunks above us.

At about ten o'clock the train crew opened up the sleeping bunks. We climbed into them in a valiant attempt to catch some sleep. Besides, the cars were dark, so there was nothing else to do. The train rocked and bumped along so much that I imagined the wheels to be square-shaped, but eventually I fell asleep.

Then all of a sudden I heard a great bang and felt the train come to a screeching halt. I had been thrown out of my bunk and was piled on the floor halfway on top of Donald. Although we were at a steep angle, we found a way to pick ourselves up and managed to find the exits. My first thought, was I hurt? No, nothing was hurting me. I was able to stand even if I was at a severe angle. Everyone seemed to be OK except the man who fell from the top side; he may have a broken arm. Then we heard the fire engines and saw flashing red and white lights.

As we stumbled around in the dark trying to figure out how to get to the doors, dozens of firemen and policemen appeared at the doors. We were helped out of the cars one at a time. As I reached the front of the door I looked out, and was shocked to see the mess all around us. Donald and I inspected each other and decided we were OK after all. We walked around in a slight daze and located a phone at a gas station near the side of the tracks. We both thought we should call our mothers to let them know we were all right. The irony was that neither of our mothers knew about the accident, so we gave them something to worry about. The biggest shock was to see the four cars in front of us, over on their sides with the first two partially crushed by the impact of hitting the earth at quite a speed.

According to what we were told, a passenger train was coming in the opposite direction on our track, and apparently our trainman self-derailed our train at a switch to miss a head-on collision. Wow! What a near miss this was. I also thought how lucky it was that the Penn RR Co. put those four cars between the locomotive and our cars. We would have been crushed or thrown to the ground and probably killed, if those train cars had not been there. We were driven to the Cincinnati Hospital for examination. A few recruits stayed there while the rest of us were bused to Memphis over the next two days.

When we arrived at the Naval Air Station in Memphis the story was written up in the local papers, and we were the center of interest for a few days. By the end of the week the story of "the train crash on the way to Memphis" was forgotten news, but now our Navy adventures were about to begin.

2. Out of Boot Camp into the Brig...Almost

After eight intensive weeks of solid physical exercise we were ready to move on to more mental activities. This did not mean the complete elimination of physical programs, but they would be cut back somewhat. The most significant change in the program was no Saturday morning classes and the chance to have a weekend pass if we were not in trouble during the week. A weekend pass was good from Friday afternoon at five P.M. until Monday morning eight A.M.

Sixty hours of freedom from physical training meant no exercise program of jumping jacks and squat thrusts and all those other exercises intended to get one into the best shape possible. The ultimate goal of the physical training was to have the unlucky ones among us have the ability to sit in one of those tiny Navy fighter planes. We were training to be aerial-gunners. If I had known exactly what that meant, I probably would never have tried to convince Aunt Flora to allow Donald to join the Navy Air Force instead of the Marine Corps.

Within two weeks of arrival, we were informed of our alternatives. Our future and possibility of survival was a matter of weight. When we enlisted the Navy recruiters painted a picture of men sitting in airplanes in warm comfortable naval bases. This certainly sounded better than sitting in a foxhole. However, after we arrived we were given more details. If you weighed less than 160 pounds, you would be assigned to fighter planes or torpedo bombers.

In actual combat, the gunner sits in the rear of these little planes, with a life expectancy of less than two minutes. The gunners sat in the rear underbelly of the fighter planes or torpedo bombers (TBFs). Their life expectancy was low because even if the Japanese gunners could not take the plane down, they could still inflict severe damage to the underside of the plane itself. At the beginning of our training we learned the cynical joke that if the plane made it back to his aircraft carrier (about a one in three chance), the pilot would ask for fill-up of fuel, more ammunition and a new aerial gunner.

As a result, we found ourselves in precarious circumstances. When one is in such situations, often one treats life very differently. Life became a wild and woolly time. Live and let live was the motto. Or live for today, who knows what tomorrow will bring? It was true that the war was winding down, but the men often joked that you were just as dead if you were shot on the last day as you were on the first.

Donald and I faced the struggle with the scale. Because Donald was at least 170 pounds he was certain to be assigned to a patrol plane (PBY). This type of aircraft was stationed off Jacksonville, Florida and safely patrolled the Atlantic and Pacific coasts. On the other hand, I weighed about 155 pounds and would probably be assigned to a TBF, the most dangerous of all assignments. This type of plane was assigned to aircraft carriers in the Pacific conflict against the Japanese, with an excellent chance of getting shot out of the sky in an engagement time of those infamous two minutes.

I remember the first day that we were given the weight versus assignment information; we decided not to tell either of our mothers. While Aunt Flora would be relieved, my mother would be devastated. We still needed about six months of training and recognized that so much could happen in that time.

But for the moment we had our first three-day pass and we were determined to have a good time. There must have been about ten of us going to Memphis for the very first time. The Navy supplied one of those antiquated school buses painted in a sickly blue color to drive us back and forth to the city of Memphis. I remember my first southern shock as we drove into town. The base was at least ten miles from the city. We drove past miles of rundown shacks the likes of which I had never known. I had never seen poor minority squalor before.

Do people actually live that way? I thought to myself. I sat with my face glued to the window taking in these horrendous scenes. I was in complete shock. I asked the man sitting next to me the same question, as I pointed to some wooden crates nailed together.

"Are you kidding? Of course they do. Where you from anyway?" I told him I was from New York and he said he was from Georgia. I mentioned that this was my first three-day pass and he said it was his first pass too. Most of the men in our company of about two hundred were either from the south (from Georgia to Texas) or from the north (New York to Boston). The Northerners knew mathematics. The Southerners knew how to fire a gun.

Donald became friendly with a group from Texas whose last names all began with "B". Our company was divided up alphabetically. I decided to hang out with Donald (Burros) and the other "B"s since I had not gotten friendly with my fellow "W"s.

We walked around the city and along the river. It was my first look at the Mississippi River and it looked very dirty. I do not remember eating dinner, but I remember the whole group meandered into a bar for drink. Although I was slightly more than eighteen, I was less sophisticated than the rest. They all ordered a drink called Southern Comfort, which I had never even heard of before, but I said I would have the same, as did Donald.

I remember that it tasted very strong and sweet, but apparently these guys were real drinkers and sat around talking about the Navy and whether they would be going into fighter planes and be fodder for the Japs. They seemed to know a lot more about what we had signed up for, than either Donald or I. Again, I felt pretty dumb because many of them had brothers or friends in the Naval Air Force.

They talked and drank, and drank and talked. They ordered round after round in what seemed to be a minute or two apart. I sat quietly taking it all in. Donald seemed to be keeping up with them. He was a much more social member of the group than I was. While I nursed my first drink along, my new Navy friends were on their third or fourth drink. I never did like to drink alcohol very much, and this Southern Comfort stuff was not "my cup of tea."

After a while these Navy guys started to fool around and although they did not seem to be violent, they were being very loud. Memphis had been a huge Navy town since 1940, but it was also a religious city. I suppose that the town's people did not like the Navy servicemen making noise in their city.

Within minutes two big Navy men walked into the bar with white uniforms and navy blue armbands that displayed two impressive letters, S.P. Everyone knew immediately whom they represented; they were the Shore Patrol. I do not believe that the guys on pass really thought that they were doing anything wrong. But I guess they did not know how strict the S.P.s in Memphis could be.

Before I knew it, they started taking the new recruits into the paddy wagon in the front of the bar. They were taken two by two and although I was rather far from the activity, I did not "look" like I was one of them. The third group included cousin Donald who seemed to be having fun with the whole scene. I walked out of the bar after this third group, and nobody stopped me or even noticed my existence.

Outside of the bar was the paddy wagon, which by this time was filled with a half-dozen boisterous sailors. While the two S.P.s went back into the bar to round-up more sailors; I wandered over to the paddy wagon whose doors were casually swung ajar.

I do not know what made me do it, but I pulled one door fully open, and discovered my cousin Donald sitting on the bench and laughing at the whole scene. Now I did not see the humor in the whole thing, but in a flash I stepped in to grab Donald and said, "let's get out of here."

I must have sobered him up with my tone, because in a second he was on his feet and out of the van while running down the street for all we were worth. Towards the end of the block I turned around to see no one following us. Boy, that was a relief!

We walked about one-half mile until we finally saw the blue Navy buses that transported the sailors back and forth to the Navy Air Station. We were finally safe.

We got on a practically empty bus because no one goes back on a Friday night. No one that is, except someone who just came out of a paddy wagon.

Monday morning at 8 a.m. those eight guys were back in the base ready to start school again. They told Donald that they spent the weekend in the brig and said it was not much fun.

3. Wrestling with Pneumonia

The Basic Navy Training Program coincidentally started on my eighteenth birthday. It was the year 1944 and the Second World War was advertised to be in its final stages. It was just one month before the most tragic battle of the war, called the Battle of the Bulge. Now in my senior years I realize that our country has a unique way of wishful thinking that its wars are over long before they actually are.

My cousin Donald and I were among two hundred sailors beginning our basic training. From there we would be programmed into one of several specialties: mechanics, radio gunners or pilot training. Pilot training involved an enlistment of four years, whereas the other two specialties required only two-year programs. We both opted for the radio gunnery program because no one really knew how long the war would actually last. It seemed prudent to volunteer for the least commitment. I actually preferred the mechanics school, but since Don was signing up to become a radio gunner, I decided to stick with him.

Basic training was a sixteen-week program followed by a four-month secondary aircraft school. The days were full from 8:00 A.M. to 5:00 P.M. We spent two hours listening to Morse code, and then the days were filled with other subjects like aircraft identification (friendly and enemy), gunnery school, where we learned how to fire .50 caliber machine guns. We took survival training courses in order to learn what plants to eat if we were ever shot down over the jungle. They also taught us to read semaphore flags and Navy signal flags, both were obsolete forms of communication, but the Navy trainers felt we should learn them in the event we would ever have to fight World War I again.

Afternoons were spent with an extremely strenuous physical training program. There were obstacle courses to run and five mile long marches. There were gymnastics, calisthenics and wrestling almost every day. At the end of the day we finished ready to collapse on our cots. Although I found the program physically challenging, I was able to keep up for the first two months. Then a circumstance occurred that in retrospect changed my entire life.

During the tenth week there was a wrestling competition among men in my company of similar size and weight. I won my first match against a man of my size and the next day I was scheduled to go against another who also won his bout the day before. We went into the ring and in about ten seconds, I was laid out flat. I had absolutely no strength, almost as if my body had lost all its power. I knew something was very wrong. Normally I was much stronger than I was that day. What was going on, I thought? Maybe I was coming down with something, so I went to the infirmary to get checked out. A nurse took one look at me, took my temperature and immediately called a doctor. Then, they took it again. I was running a temperature of 104 degrees. The nurse said, "No wonder you had no strength to wrestle" after I told her about my wrestling difficulties.

I was taken to the Navy Hospital in Memphis and given a whole battery of tests and X-rays (this was in the days before MRIs and CAT scans). The next day I was told I had pneumonia. In those days the cure for pneumonia was to drink plenty of fluids and get lots of bed rest. My temperature remained constant between 104 degrees and 105 degrees. I was a pretty sick guy. I was given cold compresses and bathes to get the temperature down.

On the fourth day the doctor came in and informed me about a new medicine just coming out of its experimental stage, called penicillin. "It is ideal for your condition," he said. That night I took an antibiotic for the first time. The next day my fever started to break and within a week I was walking around the hospital. I recuperated in the hospital over the next several weeks.

By the time I returned to the base I could no longer stay with the rest of my class, including my cousin Donald, because I had missed too many weeks of training. Just as I was going back into training, my original company, including Donald, graduated from radio gunnery school. He was assigned to patrol aircraft out of Jacksonville, Florida because of his weight. The men weighing less than 160 pounds were sent to San Diego, California for assignment to aircraft carriers and the dangerous fighter plane squadrons.

I was scheduled to go back to radio gunnery school the following Monday. On my last day at the hospital I saw a technical training program listed on the bulletin board, called the Eddy Program. The next week I took the test and was accepted into the program and again the entire direction of my life was changed. The Eddy Program was named after Captain Eddy who originated it. It was probably one of the most important programs established by the Navy to affect the outcome of the war. The program would develop a cadre of technicians who would be able to overhaul and repair the latest electronic devices entering the Navy's fleet. Of course, the equipment would become known as radar.

I entered the Eddy program in the spring of 1945 instead of completing the radio gunnery training and being squeezed into fighter planes with a mortality rate I did not even want to think about. The program was the most interesting and challenging one I ever took and included going to three schools in Chicago and Detroit over a period of eighteen months. I no longer needed to learn obsolete signal flags or run two-hour obstacle courses. This training involved working on the latest in microwave tubes and wave guide elements. It was all state-of-the-art stuff and I loved it.

After I completed the program I stayed on to teach in the program itself. In 1946 when I was discharged from the Navy and applied to Brooklyn Poly to reenter their engineering school. I was given the opportunity to continue with my original major of Chemical Engineering or switch to Electrical Engineering. One big advantage in switching majors was that I would be given sixteen credits for the work I did in the Navy's Eddy program. I made the decision to switch to the electrical program since I already loved electronics. From that point forward the direction of my professional career was changed. I have often thought about the way my bout with a little bacteria germ affected my entire life.

4. A WINTER AT NAVY PIER AND THEN SOME

We arrived at Chicago's Navy Pier in November of 1945. From the day we arrived, the weather was as bad as any winter I ever experienced in New York. It was one of the coldest winters on record. To make matters worse, Navy pier is about one mile out into Lake Michigan; when the wind blows from the Lake toward the pier it is as brutal as it gets anywhere in the country. There were about six hundred students living and learning on the pier. In six months one is prepared to maintain some of the most sophisticated equipment in the fleet.

One of the most difficult problems was to teach potential technicians to respect the damagers of high power and high voltage. On top of each piece of radar equipment was a picture of a sailor with his fingers scarred to the bone. The instant you saw that picture you did not have to be told to keep your fingers away from the output tube or the high power antenna. It was a difficult picture to look at, but it taught you a valuable lesson very quickly. Our training began at 8 A.M. and continued until 4 P.M. five days a week. We learned complex material at a rapid pace. It was the equivalent to two years of college courses in Electronic Engineering.

After the classes and laboratories we had two hours of study, and every third night we had a guard duty assignment or other work. The most unpleasant one was guard duty at the lake end of the pier. Four of us would walk around the end of the pier looking for invaders. It was no joke that the Navy commanders believed that the pier had to be protected from possible invasion from the north. We would need to stand at the edge of the pier in the outdoors with winds of twenty to thirty miles an hour in temperatures of zero or below. Every two hours we were allowed to come in to warm up. We stood around the little belly stove, drank some horrible tasting coffee, told each other how hard the work was, and complained about the ludicrous nature of each assignment.

Every other weekend we got a pass to be able to go off base into Chicago. During WWII Chicago was considered to be the best liberty town in the whole country, and we took full advantage of the chance to have a great time. Chicago had this reputation because it had wonderful facilities for sailors. An entire building near Lincoln Avenue and Congress Avenue was dedicated to the needs of the service man. There were bowling alleys, eating facilities, dance halls and libraries. Even if you wanted to be alone, there were places to go. If you wanted to meet others there were places to socialize. It was just a wonderful place for a young nineteen-year-old sailor away from his home for the first time.

One day I was surprised to hear that a good friend from Belle Harbor had enlisted in the Navy. Allan Mirkin was going to be stationed in the Great Lakes Naval Training Center just outside of Chicago. We started to correspond and made arrangements to meet after he was able to leave the training center. (In those days Basic Training was called Boot Camp and lasted for about eight Weeks.)

We met at the USO Service Center and I remember that it felt so good to see an old friend from back home. There was something so special about meeting this guy who began kindergarten with me some fourteen years earlier. We tried to meet every time we had weekend passes together. Unfortunately, in a month or two, Allan was transferred and I stayed in Chicago.

One thing about being in the service is that relationships are all too temporary, and before you knew it, one or both of you would be off again. After I finished my training, I was assigned to instruct new Eddy Program sailors in the fundamentals of Radar. That job only lasted for several months and one fine day I received a transfer notice to report to Lido Beach in New York. The notice indicated that I would receive an Honorably Discharge from the United States Navy. It seemed that this phase of my life was about to end. Well, maybe not quite yet.

I arrived in Lido Beach at the beginning of June and the next five weeks was a series of anticipations because servicemen were being discharged on the basis of seniority. At that time a lot of men were coming back from overseas with two and three years service. Those men were processed earlier and I would have to wait since I had been in the service for about 18 months.

As cold as Chicago had been in the winter, that was how hot New York was in the summer. No air conditioning existed anywhere on the base, so the station felt like a living furnace. I spent the most boring month of my life waiting around the base from morning until night. Day after day, week after week we waited for our names to be posted. I would have been happy to have been given KP (kitchen police) rather than do nothing. I said that later, but I may not have been happy if I was given sink loads of dishes to wash. Then, on the first of July my name was finally listed for July discharges, and my Independence Day had finally arrived. On the third of July, I took the Long Island Railroad to Penn Station and the BMT subway to my apartment in Brooklyn, where my family eagerly welcomed me home.

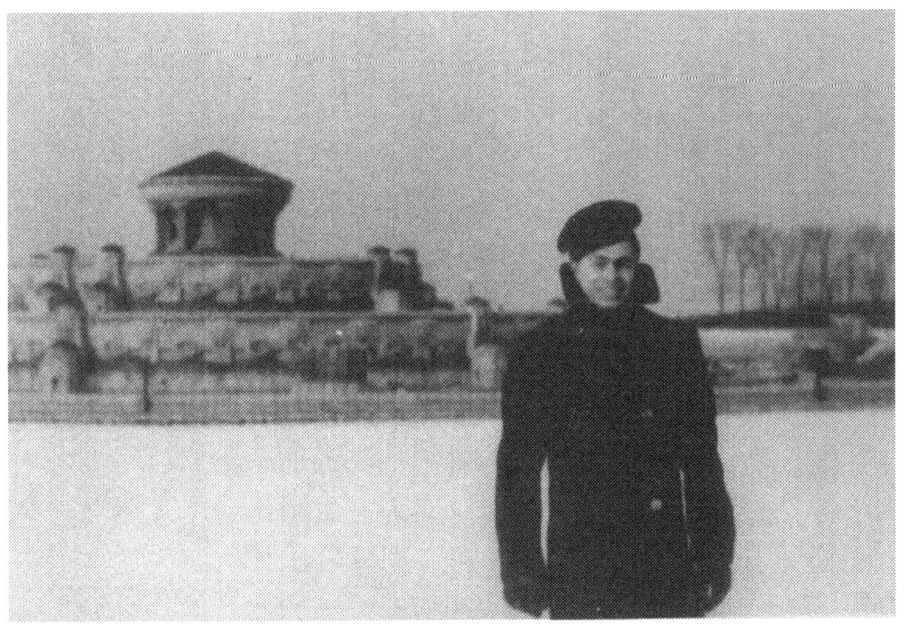

Gene in the Navy

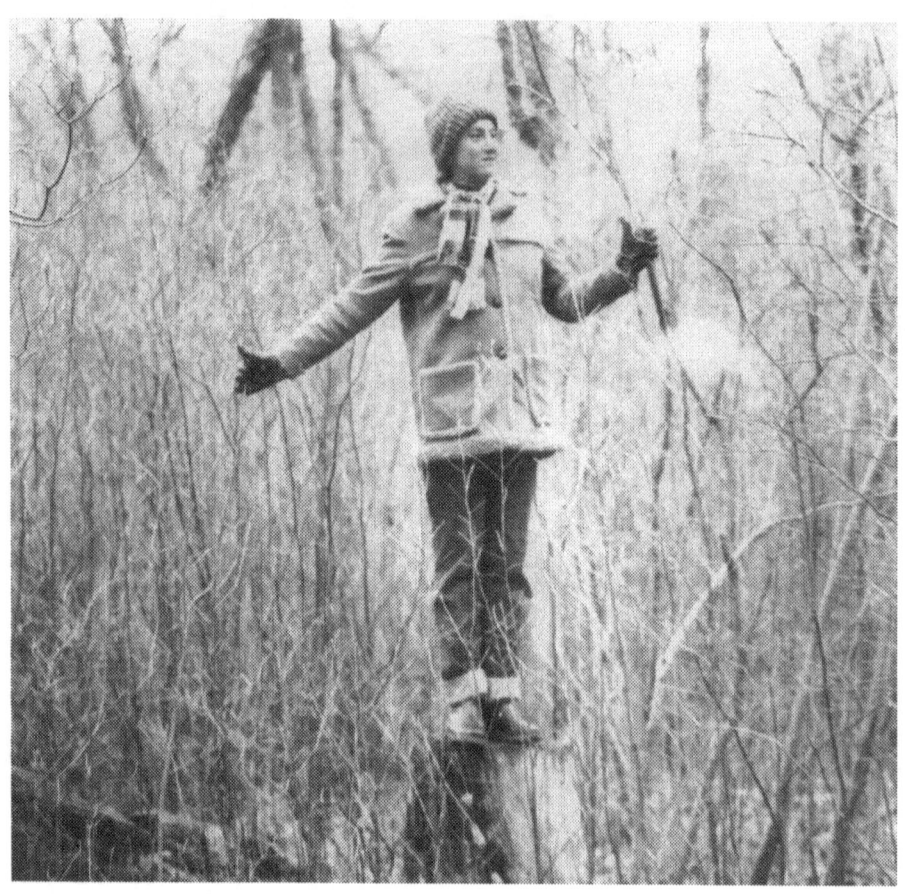

Lila Watching Gene

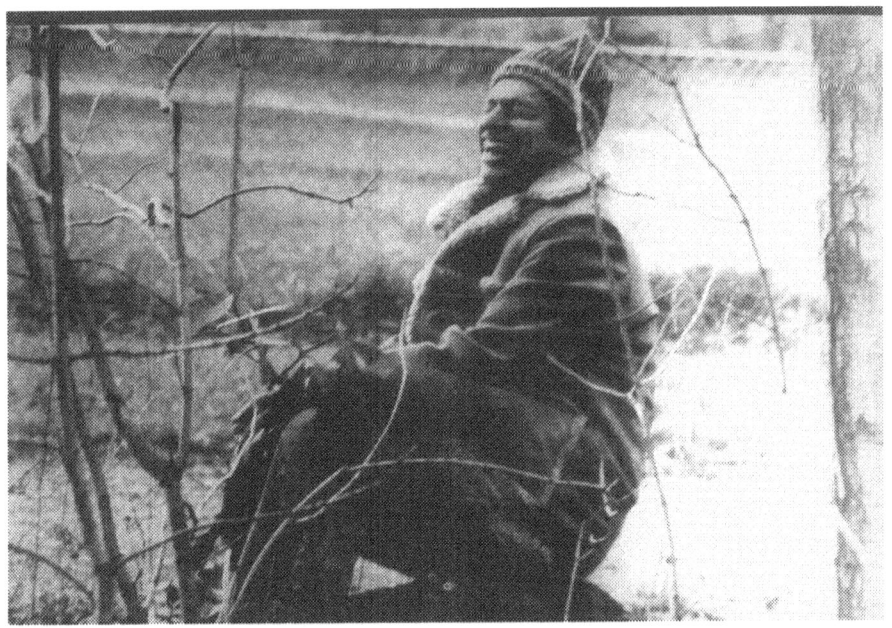

Laughing at the World

Chapter Three: My Career

Dedicated to Max Adler

1. INSIDE STORY OF BECOMING A G.M.

In 1972 I celebrated my twentieth year with the company. Gradually, I moved up from engineering into production management and from contract administration into program management. You might say I tried my hand in everything over the years. I certainly had a variety of experiences critical for general management. There was only one problem.

Moses Shapiro, the CEO of General Instrument Corporation, still remembered me as an engineer. On two occasions when GM's left our company, I was given the job temporarily and then Monty would go "to the outside" for a permanent GM.

In September 1972 Irving Kaufman suddenly handed in his resignation, and told Monty he would be leaving in three weeks.

Monty was furious, but Irv said his new company, Page Communications, wanted him there on October 1st or he would not get the job. This seemed highly unusual when filling such a high level position. In any case Irv told Monty that he had "no problem because Gene can step in and take over." In any case Monty never liked to be told anything, so he was unhappy to hear that the position was temporarily filled.

Monty called me in and told me that he was going to get someone from the outside again but "I can take over for awhile until he finds someone." Now, it was my turn to get furious. I had been the "back-up man" on two other occasions and now he was going to do it to me again. I made the decision to play hardball. I told Monty that without another job, I also would be leaving on October 1st if I could not get the position permanently.

I knew Monty could not get a replacement for me so quickly, and even if he did, there would be no one to teach him the "ropes."

The next day I told him that he had three days to make up his mind. Monty called human resources with less than two weeks to go, and begrudgingly told the representative to notify me that I got the job, but "it was not too permanent."

Over the next few months I did not hear from Monty. My only contact with him was to review the finances once a month. I did not argue with him as Irv did. I would just tell him the facts—the good and the bad. In the beginning I found out some things that were mostly bad. After reporting some rather difficult numbers, I overheard Monty telling the corporate comptroller," Now I know why Irving left so fast."

I believe that we gradually turned the business around with my determination and with a great team working together. About a dozen years after he retired Monty said, "You were the best thing I ever did for that division." I found it so interesting that he gave himself all the credit for my taking over the division and conveniently forgot the fact that I had to force him into it. But, that was Monty.

2. Works and Plays Well with Others

An important change in education took place so many years ago that one hardly ever thinks about it any more. It happened when I was a sixth grade student at P.S. 114 in Belle Harbor. Initially, students all took it with a laugh and did not take it seriously.

I brought home my report card for my mother to sign, and said something like, "Look Mom, we get a mark for playing now." For years a report card only indicated your abilities by subject studied, a B for English, A for History, A for Geography, A for Arithmetic and so on. Then, a sea change took place; on the backside of the new card were four new items for grading. I do not remember three of them, but the one that stuck with me for all these years was given the descriptive name, "Works and plays well with others."

Some thought this long sentence would never get attention from parents. Would they notice the difference between marks for individual subjects to a description of our ability to get along with others? People rarely pay attention to such a long statement. But it went from a laugh to a very important consideration for both students and parents. Sixty years later I still think about how important those six words meant in the evaluation of ones ability to get along in the outside world.

It took me over forty years to rediscover the significance of getting along with others and I would like to share it through this story. Twenty years ago when I was General Manager of the Radio Receptor Division of General Instrument Corporation, a staffer suggested there be added education for division management. He recommended we all take a management course at the AMA (American Management Association). I signed up for one of twenty courses offered at the AMA beginning the next month. It was an intensive one-week management course with about a dozen others.

I was confident that I knew most of the material because, after all, I had completed an MBA graduate program at New York University and Hofstra in the late nineteen fifties. Nevertheless, I stuck with it because it was a great review of management techniques, and I found the instructors very interesting. On the fourth day we were divided into four groups of six each, and were given the topic of working out a merger depending on our analysis.

On Wednesday evening we were given a whole set of data to study, in order to prepare a presentation regarding the merger on Thursday. The six of us were supposed to be a board of directors trying to determine whether or not to merge with another company in our business. We were given a full bill of particulars about our company, as well as information about the company we were considering for the merger.

On Thursday we spent the better part of the day analyzing the pro and cons of merging, and what share of the market we would ultimately conquer if we did merge. We also considered what products we could continue and what plants we would close or keep open, etc. It was a challenging day because we worked really hard on the project. On Friday morning we were informed that there was pending discussion regarding the merger. All of us expected that this part would be an evaluation of the various aspects of the merger.

However on Friday morning one of the members of the team introduced himself as an industrial psychologist. His goal was to analyze the behavior of the members of the group, and not the results of the merger. In effect, the real issue was an evaluation of how well each of us got along with the others to achieve the best results. His conclusion about my style was that I had the best ideas for the resulting merger, but I was far too aggressive in getting them across. He felt I had to work harder to listen to the other group members, and not be so pushy with my ideas.

I was shocked to hear that I was so aggressive. After all, was I not the one who believed in working and playing well with others? I spent the whole weekend thinking over what I had learned during the training.

On Monday morning at my regular staff meeting, I told my staff about the course. However, instead of writing down what I heard, I asked my team members for their frank opinion of my management style. I asked them to tell me honestly, without recriminations, did I do what the psychologist said I did?

I looked around the table in complete shock because slowly almost everyone began to nod their heads in agreement. Obviously, I had been a lot more aggressive than I ever thought. What a learning experience that was! I suddenly realized that I did not work and play as well as I thought.

From then on, I always tried to listen to the reaction about my ideas, instead of being aggressive about getting them out. What a learning experience that turned out to be. During the next ten years I tried to be more of a listener and less of a lecturer. I think it worked because throughout the years, many of the employees expressed that I became a better manager after that.

3. LEAD BY EXAMPLE

I had been working at Radio Receptor for several years now when there were rumors around the company. I was a young hard-working engineer, my morals were impeccable, and was raised in a family of honesty and integrity. One worked for his pay and I never knew any other way.

These rumors were disturbing to my moral code. Was it possible that they were true? Could people be taking money from vendors to place orders with certain companies instead of others? Could purchasing agents actually be doing such things?

My department was responsible for approving products from vendors. There were hints that certain companies were being chosen for reasons other than price, delivery and performance. Was I hearing correctly? Were the junior engineers and technicians telling me things that if true, were shocking to my ears?

I was in an ideal position to approve or disapprove certain vendors' parts. My components laboratory group leader, a very honest, young Chinese engineer, Frank Chin let out a hint. He heard a rumor about someone taking some money. I did not want to know. Was he asking me if I knew or if I was interested in participating? Just what was he saying? The reason I mention that he was Oriental is because sometimes people from the Far East have a way talking about things in roundabout ways. Nevertheless, I made it very clear that the only way I would approve products was on the basis of their performance. It was his responsibility to report every bit of data in an accurate way. I made this very clear, and there would be no two ways about it.

I was never approached from any sources myself. An engineer outside my department told me that some of the purchasing agents were getting kickbacks from certain chosen vendors. It was shocking when one man asked me directly if I was involved! My answer was a definite, "No way!" This question informed me that for one, he was not involved or else he would not have asked me, and second, that it gave more evidence to the rumor that it was probably happening in the company. I went to my laboratory engineer again to ask him directly if he had been approached by anyone. He assured me that he had not been directly asked to do anything like that. His answer was good enough for me.

But I was not naive enough to know the old adage, "Where there is smoke there is fire." Something else was going on these rumors were true. In a short time another rumor cropped up like poison ivy in a flower garden. The angry production engineer from my car pool was apparently let go for poor performance. This man said that he knew that scrap metal was being sold in the machine shop to a company that was owned by one of our managers.

First, it was one thing, and then another and now another, and I did not like it. It became clear to me that there were a lot of illegal practices happening in our company. In a rather short period of time, we were surprised to hear that General Instrument was buying Radio Receptor for a bargain price. Several department heads were laid off and Ralph Mendel, who had the reputation of being completely honest, became General Manager and the old GM was out.

During my first twenty years at the company I saw two very different styles of business integrity. One approach is where management's eyes are closed to kickbacks and payoffs, where illegal things are done to get money into the hands of middle management or even worse, the higher-ups. This is the type of deceit that has been happening throughout the United States, but is finally being exposed in the past few years. Often it has led to the companies' downfall, for example, the Enrons, Delphias, and Tycos. This fraud has existed in dozens of other companies in this country, and it often started at the top, so I believe it is necessary to change management.

When Ralph Mendel took over General Instrument/Radio Receptor, the rumors and intrigue quietly disappeared. I knew things were going to be different and it remained this way throughout the years Ralph was in charge. As soon as I became a General Manager I knew what type of leader I wanted to be. I wanted my employees to see by example that a reputation of honesty and integrity starts at the top. I knew that if I wanted them to be honest, that it would begin with the tone I set. There are no ifs, ands, or buts, one leads by example. There is no other way!

And so, during the generation that I was General Manager and President of my organization, there was nothing illegally taken by employees. Of this I am justly proud.

4. "Knowing where my cable went": My Proudest Program

One of my most significant leadership qualities was the ability to motivate our employees. Over the years I felt that improving employee morale through innovation and caring was an important function of a General Manager. Here is an example.

Our division received a very important contract in the late 1970's for the design, production and installation of an Electronic Warning System for the U. S. Navy's P-3B Patrol Aircraft. Our engineers and programmers worked day and night to meet a difficult nine-month schedule. In addition to the engineering, assembly and test effort, we also had to install and cable the aircraft to be ready for the flight test program.

As the time for delivery drew near we found that the Navy intended to fly the plane overseas for the test. They planned to fly the aircraft up north from Patuxient River Naval Air Base to New York to make it possible to do some final test in our area.

One day I had the idea to bring some of the engineers and programmers out to MacArthur Airport to see the plane. Then, I expanded the idea to include all the workers on the program to give them the opportunity to see the results of their labor. I thought it would be great for the morale of those who worked so hard on the project. Although it was going to be quite an effort, I felt it was worthwhile.

One evening I mentioned the idea to my family, when someone said, "How do you know who worked on it?" This question made me realize how difficult drawing that line was going to be. The next morning I called Frank Hickey's office to get permission to take the entire division to view the P-3B aircraft at MacArthur Airport. I also decided to call the Corporate Controller for approval since this task now involved a much greater expense and possibly added liability insurance.

The next day I received a call from Frank Hickey, Corporate CEO. "What's this all about?" he questioned. I explained that the P-3B program was very important to our division and we had an extremely tight schedule and that our people had been working very hard on the project. Finally, I told him that this was an idea in motivating workers. Frank seemed interested because he was concerned with improving employee morale.

On the spur of the moment, I said, "Frank, this would be a great time for you to meet many of our employees. Why not come out with Steve Davidson (VP of Human Resources)?" There was a long silence. It was typical of Frank to think through ideas slowly. I knew not to disturb his thought process while it going on. The silence seemed endless.

Finally, I knew he was in agreement, when he asked, "What time would we have to be there?"

"Oh!" I said, and the first thought that came to mind,

"Eleven o'clock, Frank, so we could tie it in with lunch." It was later that I asked myself, what did I say? Lunch for five hundred is no longer small change.

The next thing I received approval for was sandwiches and drinks for the entire division, in addition to ten buses. Of course, members of the Navy flight crew, our key employees and Mr. Hickey, and my staff had a special luncheon at a local restaurant at the conclusion of the ceremonies. In addition to company approval, it was necessary for us to obtain U. S. Navy and Islip MacArthur Airport complex approval. But after some effort, everything was finally lined up.

The day came and ten buses left our plant on a bright fall morning for one of the most impressive days I can remember. True to his word, Frank arrived with Steve at the airport to greet almost five hundred workers with a smile and warm words. His dignified six foot six inch frame and booming voice impressed many of the workers, some of who had never seen him before.

As the buses left our plant, in Hicksville for the airport, the P-3B left Patuxient River Naval Air Station in Maryland with a crew of dedicated Navy officers and enlisted men that included Lt. Commander Chuck Jeffries, Master Chief Larry Veray, and Senior Chief Tony Land. The General Instrument staff included Joel Morris, Ron Myer, Dennis Larock and Judy Halperin, who had been working so hard to complete the program on time. There were so many others, but it is now difficult to remember all of them. As Tony Land, who joined General Instrument after the initial program, said recently, "I am getting too old to remember everybody's name."

I watched as lines of workers passed through the aircraft to see our equipment including receivers, computers, cables and antennas that had been extraordinarily installed. As I stood beside the antenna and cable installation, I overheard two women production workers talking to each other.

> "I saw where my cable went and it looked great," one said.
> "There is a box I put together under a bench," said another.

"This is the first time I ever saw anything I ever built on a plane before. This is fun." remarked yet another worker.

Ron Myer, the project manager of the GI equipment told me many years later that he too remembered hearing similar comments. "All the workers were tremendously impressed," he said at a recent GI reunion. The ten man Navy crew, including officers and enlisted men in their working uniforms, came out of the plane to take pictures with the systems engineers and programmers. It was an impressive sight and one could see that they were all having a lot of fun. No fancy uniforms or white hats because it was a working day for everyone.

At the end of the excursion, the company workers got back into the buses and returned to the factory with a new and valuable understanding of our product. Afterwards the Navy officers and enlisted men joined in a celebration lunch with Mr. Hickey, my staff and the project people who worked so hard for nine months.

For me and for so many others, it was a day we will never forget. During the next five years we made many generations of this equipment for P-3 aircrafts, each generation of electronic warfare system designed to be better than the previous one. After the United States Navy program, we also made systems for Japan, Norway, and Spain among others.

I am forever in debt to all the people who worked so long and hard on that program. In my thirty-nine year career with General Instrument I believe this program was the most successful, and the one that I feel made me most proud. To think it all began with a high-pressured nine-month schedule culminating on the tarmac at MacArthur Airport in Islip, New York and a little lady finding her cable in the big P-3B aircraft.

Yes, there were engineers, programmers, program managers and technicians that worked directly on the program, but it was that unknown lady who represented all the others that were vital to the success of the program.

As I write this story a generation after that success, I have thought whether to include a list of all the people who were instrumental to the program. If I were to mention scores of names, but leave out one or two, those people would feel justifiably upset. So, I ask that everyone who participated accept my heartfelt thanks for making it a program we can all feel so very proud.

Here are some responses from others:

Judy Halperin writes:

> I, too, remember that day well, as I was on the flight back from Pax. Funny however, that the first thing that came to mind in remembering that day was the picture we all had of one of the Navy guys (maybe Chuck Jeffries or Tony Land?) "mooning" us from the cockpit while we had our photos taken standing in front of the plane below!!! Maybe some of the other readers would remember that, too...
>
> What a wonderful response to your e-mail by Ron Myer. I think that he captured the sentiments of all of us who worked at GI during those years. For many of us it was the best working experience we've had, and that particular project truly embodied the meaning of teamwork!!

Joel Morris writes:

> Your story does recap some wonderful memories of a time I also am most proud. There is another aspect that you may find interesting as well. Our staff, as you know, was working very hard to make the flight test successful. We were informed of your intentions to bring the entire company out to meet us as we landed at Islip airport. As you may remember one of the key objectives was to perform a precision DF (Direction Finding) measurement, which we were not able to achieve. In Patuxient River, we had a last flight test, before we were to fly to Islip. On that last flight Dennis Larock found that the servo to the radar antenna was miswired, i.e. two wires were reversed. We corrected the error, and viola! we obtained the precision DF measurements.
>
> We all thank Dennis for his efforts as the in-house coordinator and also for Irv Rothbloom's management of the engineering team.

5. THE BIRTH OF SEA BEAM

Each evening I would sit around the dinner table with my wife and four alert children, and often talk about the happenings at General Instrument. I was so lucky to have an exciting job to share with an interested family. Some evenings I would come home and talk about the functions of a radar warning receiver; other nights, the discussion revolved around an upcoming trip to a Defense Electronics Show in Paris.

At times I would bring home information about the undersea mapping systems. I found this project an exciting one that started with the germ of an idea from two innovative engineers, Howard Lustig and Arthur Rossoff, in our Hicksville, New York facility. Their original concept was to develop a multi-beam radar system and install it into a U. S. Air Force airplane. The aircraft would then be flown over the Soviet Union to map the contour of their territory. This happened at the beginning of the cold war, almost one-half century ago. However, the program did not continue due to circumstances that discouraged the Air Force from proceeding.

At that point we had a brilliant idea without a home. Fortunately, our ingenious engineers from the transducer facility, Don White and Harold Farr, came up with a clever variation to this multi-beam concept. Their idea was to have it used with a multi-beam sonar system. It would be installed on a ship to map the ocean bottom, instead of an airplane.

General Instrument fortuitously purchased a small division in Boston started by a sonar engineer named Wilber Harris. This division was the basis for the multi-beam system. The unit, Harris Transducer Division made projectors and receivers for the sonar industry. On a memorable day in early 1960, Howard and Arthur paid a visit to the key engineers at Harris, Harold Farr and Donald White. They discussed the possibility of using the latest in computer technology to invent a system that would be able to make real-time maps of the ocean bottom.

They approached the U. S. Navy with this extremely creative concept. After six months of proposal writing and making presentations to key Navy officials, the idea was finally funded. The Navy gave the project to a young, aggressive engineer at the Naval Material Laboratory, Steve Kochansky. Coincidentally, I had worked with Steve ten years before in the Brooklyn Navy Yard. Although I had nothing to do with the design, my relationship with Steve was helpful when the program would get bogged down.

Two years later an initial system was installed on a research ship called the Compass Island. The concept worked even though the computer was unreliable.

This system would automatically generate maps as the ship steamed along, instead of requiring dozens of cartographers to draw contour lines of the ocean's bottom. After the initial program, a new contract was funded for four additional systems called the Sonar Array Sounding System.

As these four systems were delivered during the late 1960's the ocean began to get mapped in earnest. It was now possible to get accurate detailed data of the ocean bottom. Hundreds of maps were created that made layers beneath the ocean visible to scientists and military people alike. Initially, the systems were used for highly classified projects. During the Cold War they were used to track the path and location of Russian submarines throughout the world. The U.S. Navy forbade us to discuss the concept with other nations because of the very sensitive nature of the data.

There was continued disagreement between the scientists who wanted to use the data for oceanographic purposes, and the military people who wanted the data to remain classified because of its military significance. Ultimately, General Instrument personnel convinced the Navy that if we did not sell it to other countries, they would eventually develop it themselves. It was clear that multi-beam technology was here to stay with the advent of more powerful computers.

For years there were problems with the hand drawn charts of the middle of the Atlantic Ocean. There were so many irregularities that the work of the cartographers was stymied. The year 1974 was designated as FAMOUS, which was symbolic for the French-American Mid-Ocean Undersea Study. It was a year dedicated to increased understanding of our ocean surfaces. The French were given the challenge of getting the mapped data about the entire middle Atlantic ridge. The French had the macro responsibility while the Americans had the micro responsibility.

The only way to see the overall bottom of the ocean surface was to use a multi-beam sonar system and General Instrument was the only company to have such a system. We were called to Paris to negotiate a contract for our system. The French were egocentric about their technical abilities and were also very sensitive about the fact that they needed to buy such technology from the United States. (General Instrument had the patent for the technology.)

The program manager, Don White, and I spent a long week in Paris trying to negotiate an agreement with their Hydrographic Office. To make matters more difficult, the office at Idlewild Airport (renamed John F. Kennedy Airport) passed a ruling that limited the number of planes allowed to land at that airport. The ruling annoyed the French even more because the U.S was squeezing Air France out of the airline market. So they were not happy about purchasing a Sea Beam from an American company. In fact, the French negotiator told me off the record that if the technology could have been bought "anywhere in the world other than the United States, they would have done so."

Although they hated us that week, we just hung in there. When I reported back to the General Manager, he said something I have quoted many times since I became a General Manager.

He said, "the art of negotiation is the art of keeping the seat of one's pants upon the seat of one's chair."

The negotiations were made more difficult by the fact that they insisted on keeping it in French, so we needed the contract translated line by line. We later discovered over dinner and a few bottles of wine, that the French negotiators were instructed to give us a hard time. We all laughed about this, and a while later we had our contract.

For years, two divisions worked on this multi-beam sonar system. The Hicksville division worked on the electronics, while the Boston division worked on the sonar portion of the system. Because this was a very sophisticated and highly classified project, I always had to be careful not to release any classified material. Typically, I would tell others the name of the system (Sonar Array Sounding System) and that it was used to find things in the bottom of the ocean, like treasures. I never actually said anything about its real purpose.

Years later the security classification was downgraded and our company received permission to sell comparable systems to friendly foreign governments. The U.S. government insisted that the system sold overseas should be significantly downgraded in performance.

In order to separate the high performance system used by the United States Navy (referred by its complicated name, Sonar Array Sounding System or SASS) from the commercial version, we decided to create a new name. General Instrument was looking for a catchy name that distinguished itself from the Navy's, but that was also descriptive of its function. At that time, both the electronic and sonar portions of the commercial version were being built in Boston. I visited the Boston facility once a month to check on its progress.

One night after a monthly trip to Boston, I told my family that the project managers of the commercial version of SASS were looking for a new name. This task fascinated my kids and they started to ask questions about the systems' function. I explained how the system worked under the ocean to send many sonar beams to the ocean floor. After several minutes on the subject, the kids started to throw out suggestions. Among the many suggestions one potential name was Ocean Mapper and the other was Sea Mapping System. Suddenly, our youngest son who was nine years old, but very good with words, came out with the name SEA BEAM. Immediately the others repeated "Sea Beam, yes that sounds good. Sea Beam! Yes!" They said, "That sounds good." And so Sea Beam was born.

We delivered the Sea Beam to the French in time to meet the "1974 Year of Exploration" and several of our engineers were there to use the system in the mid-Atlantic. They returned with stories about what they found. In the middle of the Atlantic we saw a huge gully that was later called the Mid-Atlantic Ridge. It was this data that showed that the plates under the ocean were actually separating causing Europe and North America to move apart.

Over the next forty years hundreds of scientific discoveries were made possible with the use of Sea Beam. Sea Beam systems were delivered to Australia, Japan, Korea and others. Eventually, our patent ran out and the French and Germans started to manufacture Sea Beam type systems. But the name Sea Beam began at a kitchen table when a young boy thought of a catchy name for this very important system.

6. MY MOST MEMORABLE MOMENT

Looking back at the days before this particular seminar, I remember there was great concern about whether or not I was going to be healthy enough to attend. Never before did Steve seem so concerned about my attendance at the seminar. It was the year 1983 and in the five years since Frank Hickey became CEO, we always had these Executive Management Training Weeks in interesting places. However, this year it was being held close to the corporate headquarters in New York.

When Moses Shapiro was CEO we never had out-of-town sessions. During Shapiro's tenure we would have one-day meetings at the corporate offices in New York with Shapiro spending the majority of time as the star. Under Frank's leadership we would get together out of the city and spend a week with professional trainers conducting seminars, group discussions and social get-togethers, in addition to reviewing the financials.

The previous year we met in Phoenix, Arizona; which is one of Frank's favorite places. On the last night we all got together in an old western town where they had an old-fashioned cowboy shoot-out following cattle drive through the center of town. I think Frank enjoyed them even more than the rest of us.

Frank loved the camaraderie after the business sessions. He seemed to have a dual personality. At the business meetings he was a tough, no nonsense boss, but then he liked to act like "one of the boys" after he had a few drinks. I liked him better the second way because he was warm and caring. He would say "We Jews and Irish Macs had a lot in common." He would give me a big bear hug, and be very outspoken and uninhibited as he wrapped his six-foot, six-inch two hundred-fifty pound frame around this little five-foot-eight inch one hundred-sixty pound guy. In those minutes he was a fatherly type where one could overlook his flaws, so much I would almost forget the hard time he gave me in the auditorium six hours before.

Fortunately during most of my tenure as GM my division's performance was above average, so I rarely knew the discomfort of his wrath. His comments about me were often "You are the most unsupervised General Manager in the company." In general he was very satisfied with our division's performance. There is one instance I will always remember that showed our relationship and our personalities.

During one annual review after I made an especially effective presentation, I asked for an additional three million dollars for capital expenditures. He thought it over for several long, hesitant minutes. At long last he said, "OK, I will take some of your snake oil." In a way his remark was a compliment, but at the same time showed his skepticism. I took his comment with a smile and went back to my division headquarters with the wonderful news that our request for additional funds had been accepted. As usual we worked hard and effectively all year long. The resultant year was one of our best and I was felt exuberant.

As the fiscal year came to an end and we were planning for the annual presentation, I thought of a great idea. I must have felt somewhat insulted with his "snake oil" remark, so in a very subtle way I attacked him in an area of his vulnerability, which was drinking. Everyone knew that Frank had a strong drinking habit. He was not an alcoholic, but did love to drink. I decided to buy him a bottle of his favorite scotch, Chivas Regal. Giving him a bottle at the annual business meeting would have meant nothing, aside from a small insult, but it was what I had done with the bottle that mattered. I had our artist relabel the bottle from the picture of the Scotchman dressed in a kilt to a drawing of a snake with the encircled words, "Gene's Elixir of Snake Oil."

As the meeting began, Frank took the package graciously and put it aside. But that was not good enough for me, and I insisted he open it right then and there. Finally Frank concurred, unwrapped the package, looked at the label, immediately remembered his remark the previous year about trying some of my "Snake Oil" and roared with laughter. When he stopped laughing, all he could say, "Gene, you are something else!" Frank and I certainly had a wonderful relationship during our twenty-five years, but this was one of the highlights.

Three months later as we prepared for a general managers session, this time in New Jersey, I had a physical condition that required immediate surgery. I was absent for about two weeks, but returned on a part-time basis before the GM program. The last week before the sessions, I received several calls from Steve Davidson, Human Resources V. P., to inquire about my health and likelihood that I would attend the following five-day session. I told him I expected to, never stopping to think that there might have been an underlying reason for his question. The company always held very thought provoking seminars, and despite a fatigue at the end of the day, I found them really exciting. Each division reviewed their results and Frank discussed the corporation plans for the coming year. During the evenings we enjoyed nice dinners, followed by all night poker games orchestrated by Lou Solomon, V.P. of Marketing. One night we went to a casino in Atlantic City where many of the executives "invested" some of their bonuses.

The last evening we always had a formal dinner when Frank would give us the annual pep talk. It had been a long and tiring week for me, with the all-day sessions, the trip to Atlantic City and the other late night poker games. I considered the possibility of passing up the final dinner and going to bed early but at the last minute, I decided to go since I was going home the next day and could sleep all weekend.

I sat quietly eating my dinner around the ten person tables. There must have been fifty of us around the room, all the G.M.s, the corporate staff and financial people. Frank and the senior V.P.s sat at the dais. When the coffee was served Frank got up and started his speech. He is a good speaker, especially after he had one or two drinks. Not enough to be over-exuberant, but enough to be more relaxed than without them. He seemed to be in a great mood.

Frank talked about the future and the spirit of the company team, and that he planned to begin an annual award to the General Manager most deserving of his ability to motivate his organization. He went on for a while and I must admit I was tired from the week's business activities, the stress of my previous physical surgery, and all of the late-night activities too. I was listening only half-heartedly and thinking about how wonderful it would be to be in bed and that the dinner should be over in a little. When Frank Hickey suddenly says, "The First Annual Award for General Instruments General Manager of the Year goes to Eugene Weisberger."

The applause was long and loud. It fortunately gave me enough time to remove the fog from my brain. I walked slowly up the dais thinking about what could I possibly say. Nothing came to my mind as I reached to shake Frank's big hand. I simply started to tear-up and began to say how much I appreciated this award and how everybody in the room was more deserving than I, then Frank took the pressure off me by reading the plaque's inscription. He wrote:

> Eugene Weisberger is awarded The First Leadership Award as General Instrument General Manager of the year 1983.
>
> Gene has excelled in planned fiscal performance, in steadfast dedication to the well-being of our corporation as well as that of the division, in the delivery of advanced technology, in a market he understands, in the continuous commitment to high product reliability and beyond all else in the motivation of the people throughout the Government System Division.

Then, in my unique ability of ad libbing with a sense of humor, I started my short talk heard for years around the GI world.

> "About three weeks ago I had a real physical problem. I had to be rushed to the hospital because I could not urinate. It was a terrible sensation. But finally

the doctor arrived and using some instrument or other got me to be able to urinate again. What a relief! It felt so good to be able to go again."

I broke down the house with a remark that they will never forget. I said, "Next to being able to urinate again, this is the most memorable moment in my life."

I sat down to a resounding laughter and applause, the likes of which I had never heard.

7. REMEMBERING MAX

A General Manager's responsibility is to his top management, the shareholders, his customers, and last, but not least to his employees.

During the latter part of the 1980's, our division was under a great deal of pressure to make deliveries on schedule in accordance with a very difficult U. S. Navy production contract.

I also experienced a difficult and emotional issue that will stay with me for the rest of my life.

Max Adler was the Vice President in charge of production for over twenty years. The man in that position was critical to making the deliveries on time and within budget. He was considered the glue that made the production department work. Max was a man who knew all the details and all elements of assembly, manufacturing and production control, which made it possible for the department to function.

Max was turning 65 in January of the year we were making these critical Navy shipments. We were under pressure to meet our financial obligations with top management and the shareholders by making those deliveries in addition to the burden of meeting the Navy schedule. Hence, we had a double incentive to make those shipments.

In December of the previous year, Max told me that he expected to retire when he turned 65. I asked him for a big favor to extend work for an additional month, until the end of the fiscal year, February 28th. The next day, he told me he would stay on as I had requested.

December and January were two difficult months for our division because our shipments fell behind by about 20 percent. It was a cold winter, and Max told me he was looking forward to going down to Florida and sitting in the warm sunshine.

It was apparent by the third week of February at our production meeting, that we would not meet the Navy's delivery requirement. Again I asked Max to stay with the company until the end of March. I told him that I really needed his help. Reluctantly, he told me that he would stay until the end of March and then go to Florida.

Despite the efforts of Max and his staff, we continued to experience technical problems where many of the systems did not meet their life tests, and would require additional testing. March went into April and the production difficulties continued. Max was working extremely hard, and it even appeared as though he was losing weight. I told him that if he worked until the end of April I would give him an extra month's salary, in addition to paying for his Florida vacation.

But at last, there would be no more extensions and Max's staff arranged his final retirement party. The dinner was set for a Friday evening toward the end of May, and over two hundred people came to say farewell to this loyal, hardworking man. Max's wife, Florence made arrangements to go to Cape Cod for his much needed two-week vacation instead of Florida because the winter was over. Florence, my wife Lila, and I sat at the head table and watched Max open dozens of presents: the last being a full set of luggage for them to use the following day for their upcoming vacation. I noticed that Max seemed to be so excited that he did not eat a drop of food.

The following Monday I went back to work as usual. I did not think it was unusual that I had not heard from Max or Florence and assumed they were busy with their vacation and would call me when they returned.

Three weeks later I received a call from Florence saying that she had some bad news. Florence and Max never arrived at Cape Cod because Max was in a hospital in New York City. The day that they were going to Cape Cod, Max went to Beth Israel Hospital instead because of severe stomach pains. Just a few days after his retirement started, Max had an operation for stomach cancer.

It was such a shock to me to hear that this wonderful good friend, and great employee who had sacrificed so much for the company and me was suddenly at death's door. I felt so guilty that I had persuaded him to stay on and on with General Instrument, instead of enjoying his last few months.

Max died in August just three months after he retired at the age of sixty-five and one-half.

Max's sad ending reminded me of an Oscar Wilde fable, "The Happy Prince" that I vaguely remember from my early years. The story may not be accurate, but I think that it expresses my thoughts about Max's situation.

The Happy Prince

A wonderful statue of a Prince sat in the center of a park. It was ordained with many silver and gold ornaments. A bird sat on the statue's shoulder all summer long.

Around the park there were many poor men sitting with little to do, and nothing much to eat and drink. The Prince statue could see this from his pedestal and it made him very sad. He knew that winter would be coming soon and these people would have nothing to eat. As the weather started to get cold, the statue asked the bird if he would take his sword and give it to one of the poor people in the park. The bird obliged, then each day the statue would ask the bird to take another item from him and give it to another person. After a while the bird said that he would have to fly south because the weather was getting so bad, but the statue begged him to stay yet another day.

The weather was really cold now, and the statue asked the bird to take his last eye so that still another poor person would have something to get him through the winter. This time the bird said, "I must leave for the South because it is now so cold and I will not be able to make it." But the statue responded, "Oh you must do this one last favor for me so that the last poor man sitting on that bench will not starve this winter."

As the snow came down the next morning, the town's trash men noticed the damaged statue and a dead bird on his shoulder. One of them said to the other "We will have to clean up this park in the springtime."

I think of Max as this selfless little bird that devoted himself to his boss and the company by paying the price with his life. Of course, I know I do not have the power of life or death over anyone. But I feel guilty nevertheless because Max could have enjoyed some warm months in Florida, instead of working so hard those last three months.

Being a General Manager with a heart is sometimes difficult to accept. But I would rather be like the Statue Prince who suffers the guilt and torment of those hard times, while enjoying the wonderful, happy relationships with all those great people for all those years.

8. Unusual Coincidences

Recently I felt as though a huge burden had finally been lifted from my back or that I had just come back from outer space. A major task of the last few years was finally behind me. My first book, <u>The Chinese Walking Stick</u> was finally into publication. It was a huge project to write and rewrite fifty stories. I would like to write about the process someday, but for now it felt good to have it behind me.

Last night we had our periodic General Instrument get-together; it felt great to see all the old friends. Judy told me about her son's upcoming trip to Prince Edward Island. Harry is still playing golf, and Sam who is a few years older than I, is still throwing the basketball around. I always enjoy meeting my old friends and sharing tales from the old days.

During the conversation I told one group that I was going to France the following week, and that I had sent a message to that effect to my Internet readers. I received a message from Georges DeCock who now lives in Toulouse, France asking where I was going to be. I sent him my itinerary, and by coincidence our paths would cross on July 6 in his city of Toulouse, France. I told him that I would be meeting all the old GI alumni, and he asked me to give everyone his regards.

When I mentioned his name and the planned meeting in France, one of our friends, Sam Coleman recalled another coincidence that he and Georges DeCock experienced about ten years before.

It was during the time of the Japanese P-3 Aircraft program when we had a group of Japanese students staying in Hicksville for a training course. Sam who is a great storyteller recalled how he and Georges made plans to take the Japanese students to dinner one night. It was a weekend, as Sam remembered, and they made plans to meet the Japanese students at a restaurant in Syosset at 6:00 P.M. Because the students were not there by six o'clock, Sam and Georges assumed that they must have gotten lost wherever they had spent the day, so they waited and waited. Finally, the Japanese naval officers showed up at 7:00 P.M. and of course apologized for being late.

Sam asked them questions about where they spent their day off. The Japanese students giggled with each other, which was typical behavior to show they were embarrassed. Then, they hesitated for a while. Sam interpreted this silence related to a language misunderstanding, so he repeated the question. Finally they answered that they visited the aircraft carrier, The U.S.S. Intrepid in New York Harbor along the Hudson River. Sam thought to himself that this was no reason to be embarrassed, that is, until he realized what day it was.

You see it was December 7th. The Japanese officers felt the stares of all the Americans as they watched the 45th anniversary ceremony for the bombing of Pearl Harbor. The day that would live in infamy would not be the day Japanese naval officers would feel comfortable visiting the U. S. S. Intrepid in New York.

Their blunder reminded me about the day Lila and I coincidentally visited Hiroshima, Japan. We were there on August 5th, which was the 37th anniversary of the day that the United States Air Force dropped the atomic bomb on that city. We also felt uncomfortable about being in Hiroshima on that very solemn occasion.

I think I know how those students must have felt at the Intrepid.

9. GREAT TO BE REMEMBERED

Just an hour or so from the heart of midtown Manhattan is a spectacular get away hotel in the lower hills of the Catskills called the Mohonk Mountain Resort. It is a beautiful place with lots of facilities. In the days of the hotel chains like Hilton, Radisson and Best Western, it is especially great to find a place still run by its original family. For about one hundred-fifty years the Mohonk has continually grown little by little, step-by-step in its same wonderful location. The Mohonk started out as a small wayside inn mostly catering to the businessman who needed a little shady entertainment. But during an era of morality, the inn stopped flourishing, so it was sold to a family who had the exact opposite idea of what clientele to attract.

They decided to cater to the families from New York City looking for a place for summer vacations. Five generations have run this place based upon the same philosophy of offering great food, excellent recreational facilities and comfortable accommodations. You will notice I said nothing about economical rates because it is not kind the place to go if one is trying to economize. The rooms are also big and comfortable.

In addition it provided the old-fashioned three meals a day service. Nowadays you are lucky to get a continental breakfast in most hotels. Mohonk serves three classical meals with both lunch and dinner served gourmet style. There are two dining rooms. One is a formal facility that requires men to wear jackets and ties. The other dining room is buffet-style, but no less gourmet. There are six serving stations with stylish chefs at each one. In addition to a carving station, they have specially prepared salads, a variety of fish, chicken and veal dishes, as well as variety of dishes for the vegetarian. The waiter only serves beverages and dessert. It is interesting the way dessert is presented. One walks up to the dessert station and chooses a desired dessert. Then you go back to the table to tell the waiter which dessert you chose.

I was informal enough to not want to wear jackets on the hot summer days we spent at the luxurious Mohonk. During our entire stay we chose to eat in the buffet dining room. On Sunday afternoon, as I waited to get a shrimp dish that always turned out to be delicious, a man walked up to me and said, "Gene Weisberger?" I did not recognize him, so I playfully said, "No you must have the wrong person."

He looked embarrassed and said, "Oh! You look just like someone who was my boss a long time ago."

He continued, "He was a great guy. I cannot get over it. You are a spitting image of him. But, it was a long time ago and I guess people do look alike. I am sorry to have bothered you. By the way, we worked for General Instrument. Did you ever hear of it?"

"Yes, I worked there for about forty years." I said with a smile.

"You ARE Gene Weisberger! You son-of-a-gun, I can tell by the smile."

I then admitted to him that, of course, he was right. I apologized for being deceitful and told him that I was just curious to see what he would say about me. He said that he wished that all his bosses could have been as nice as I was.

Joking with him, I said, "Can you come over to my table and tell my wife that?"

I returned to our table with my plate full of food and a smile on my face. Later on in the dinner, my old employee and his wife came over to our table and I introduced them to Lila.

He repeated how great it was to work for General Instrument. In this day and age when the CEO and other execs are getting such bad press, I thought to myself that other bosses would rather have $6,000 shower curtains than have their employees say such nice things about them.

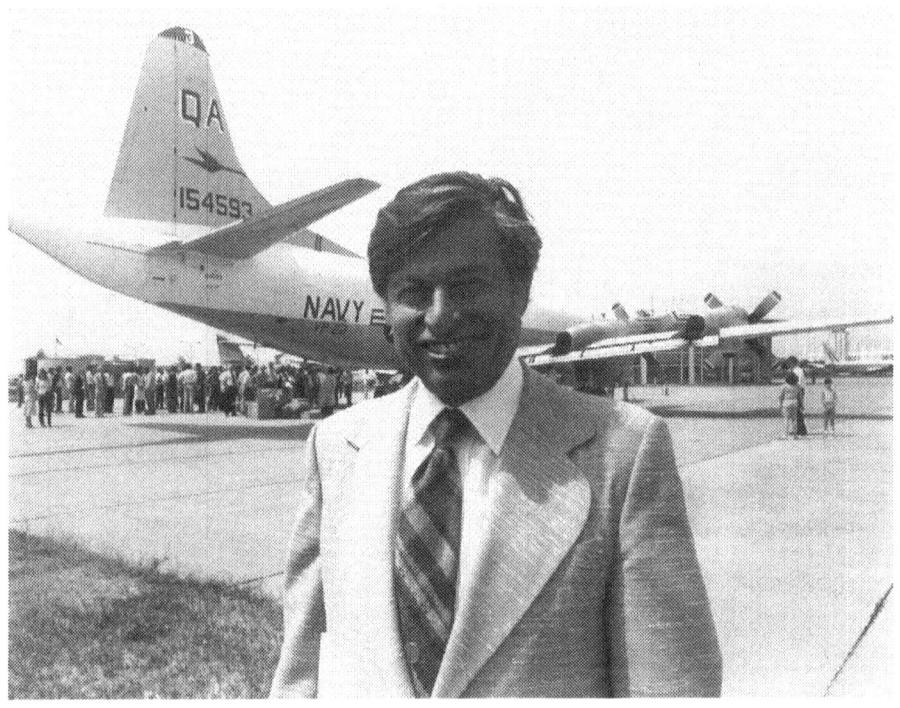

In front of Navy P-3B and Employees Lined up for Tour

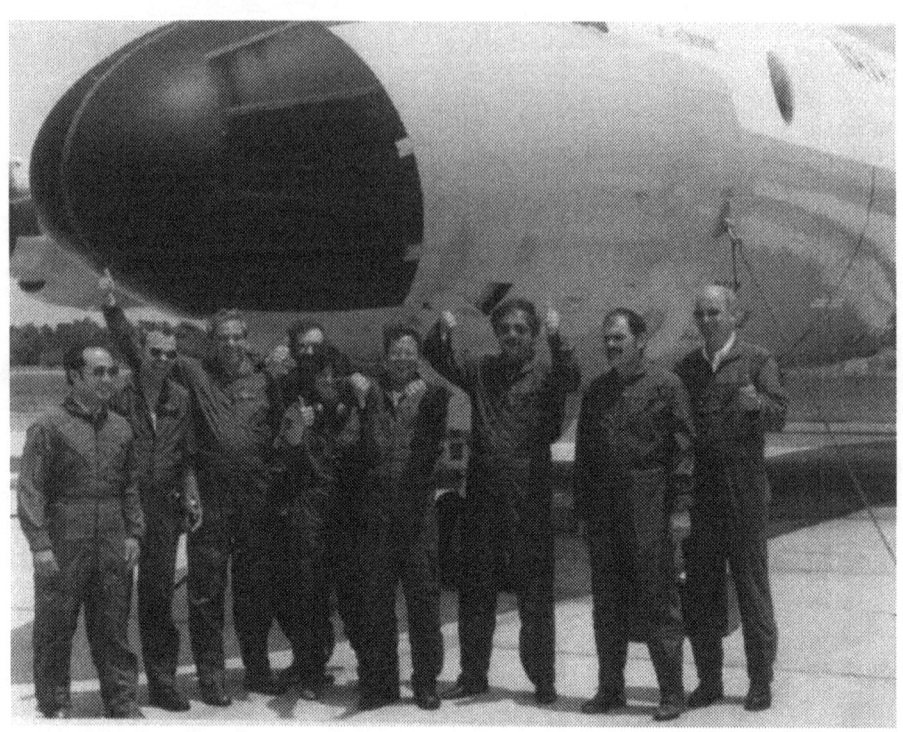

Navy and GI Crew in front of P-3B Radom

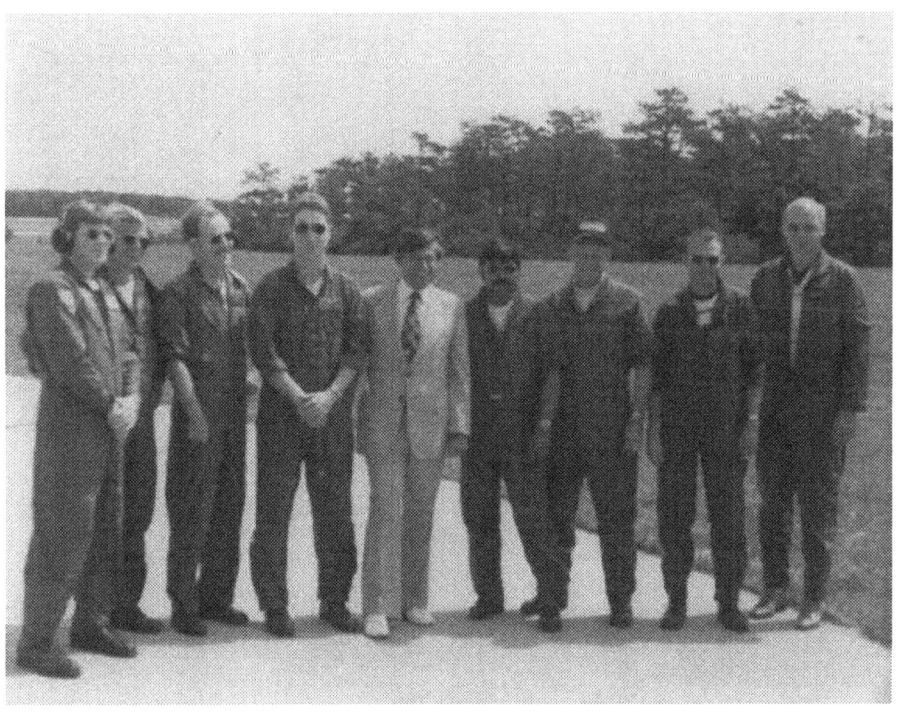

Gene with Navy and GI Team After Flight Test

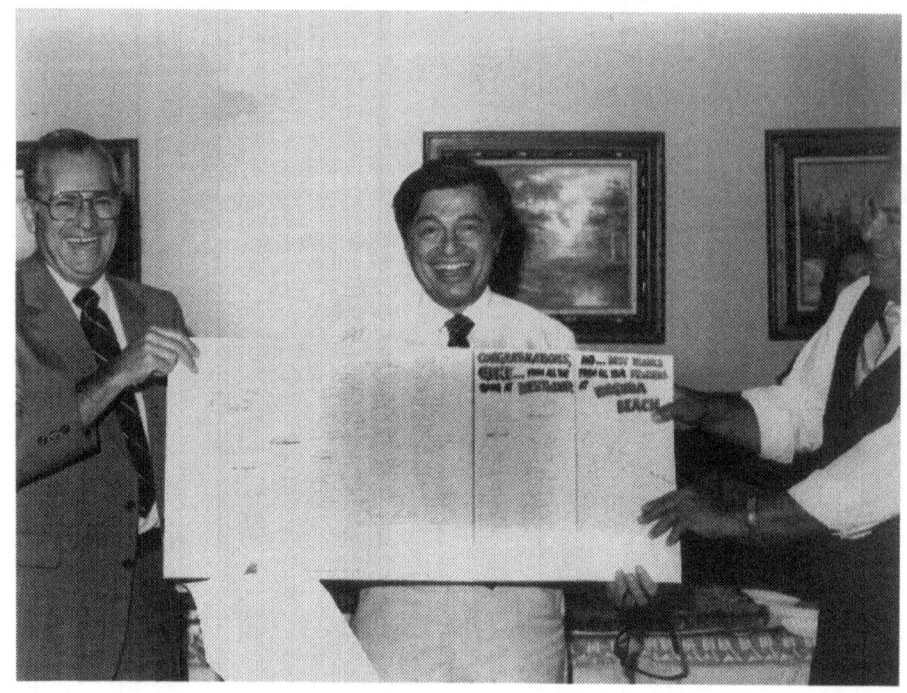

Jim Adams and Max Adler Surprising Gene

Chapter Four: The Illness

Dedicated to Dr. Mark Bilsky, Dr. Nessa Coyle, Dr. David Pfister,
Dr. Joseph Disa, Dr. Arthur Brown and the others of MSKCC Team

1. LAZARUS

A Family History Leading to Donald and Me

My first contact with Memorial Sloan Kettering (MSK) was almost synonymous with death. My closest friend and cousin in my early years was Donald. We were born just five days apart from two sisters who were as close as two sisters could be. My mother Sabina was ten years older than her sister Flora. The girls were two of twelve siblings that included eight brothers. There were five brothers between my mother and Donald's mother Flora.

My mother's job in a family of this size was to help her mother bring up all these boys. Grandma Julia was the manager of the household in addition to being the generator of offspring. When she was in her sprouting years, and was pregnant every two years for twenty, Grandma decided that my mother would be her assistant. This huge family lived in the center of Jewish life in Harlem in the early twentieth-century employed two maids. The upstairs maid did nothing but cleaning and laundry all day long six days a week. The downstairs maid did all the shopping and cooking for a dozen kids serving three meals a day, six days a week. It was an unbelievably busy household.

When my mother was eighteen years old she was expected to start college because Grandma believed that in addition to having children, women should also have a college education. Four years later my mother graduated with a teaching degree from Hunter Normal College as did her sisters.

In the household there were three children older than my mother, two girls, Annie and Nettie, and one boy, Harry. They fled the household to get married early in their life, leaving my mother the task of being the aforementioned assistant. In this incredible house of eight children younger than herself, my mother found herself raising younger seven brothers and one sister, Flora.

In 1907 tragedy struck the family and my grandfather, in his early fifties, came down with pneumonia in the time before antibiotics and died within the fortnight. Grandma did not even have time to mourn. She had to organize the family and keep the entire household from falling apart. Now she had to run her late husband's business as well as keep the household under control.

In addition to going to college each day my mother, age 19 was the main help to her mother in taking care of the children in the family. They were assisted by the older children, Abe, 17, Sam, 15, Lionel, 13, in taking care of the other children, Joe, 11, Sol, 9, followed by Flora,7, Percy,5 and Dave,3. Flora was the apple of my mother's eye, in spite of her tough girl exterior necessary for survival among this household of boys. Since grandma was so busy, Sabina became Flora's second mother.

Although my mother also finished Hunter with a teaching degree, Grandma convinced her to stay home and bring up the remaining children. She had little time to concern herself with social associations. One by one, her brothers went off to college to become lawyers and engineers.

One day as they were walking home, my mother's older siblings, Harry and Nettie, met an old friend from his school days. His name was Jacob Weisberger. Harry and Jacob walked home to the Sprung house in Harlem, and Jacob was invited to stay for dinner. The Sprung family was so big that most of the brothers did not even notice an extra face at the table.

But my mother noticed this quiet, shy young man, and in a while he was visiting Sabina more than his friend Harry. Although Grandma needed Sabina's help to raise the last three boys, she gave Jacob permission to ask for her hand in marriage in 1918.

She never stood in the way of her children's happiness.

Then my mother's little sister Flora, who also went to teacher's college at Hunter, met a hard working fellow, John Burros, and before long, she left the household to get married.

Shortly after their marriage, Flora and John had a little daughter, Elaine. Two years later in 1924, my mother and father also had a daughter, my sister, Rita. Then came 1926, which in this family would be called the "year of the grandchildren." In the span of three months, four of Grandma's children had children. Abe and Natalie's third daughter Helen was born, and Sam and Peggy had their first son, George. Then I was born in December and five days later Donald was born to John and Flora. What a prolific family!

Over the years Grandma had a total of twenty-five grandchildren, but Donald and I would become two of the closest. Not only because we had birthdays five days apart, but also because we were compatible in doing so many things together.

We spent time in day camp together. As teenagers we would become counselors at a boy's camp together. During World War II we joined the Navy together and were stationed at the same base for months.

We slowly drifted apart after we both got married and Donald moved to Washington. From time to time I would see him on a visit to Washington or when he came up to New York. Several times during our business career we planned to set up a business together. Donald sold commercial conveyor systems and I was president of a military electronics business. On two occasions we met to set up a company combining both of our operations into a joint venture, but somehow we could never raise the funds. We were quite successful individually, however, and we both lived a financially comfortable life.

We were in our early sixties when he came home one day and his wife, Marion, just knew that something was terribly wrong. Donald was the first of my cousins to be hit by a devastating form of cancer. He was admitted to Sloan Kettering for his operation. During the next few years Donald was in and out of Memorial, and I visited him on two or three occasions. But after a while he did not want me to come. This strong, vibrant wonderful man, who I had known all my life, was sadly wasting away.

Memorial Sloan Kettering was the last place where I saw him.

Memorial Sloan Kettering could do nothing to save this sweet, caring guy whom I loved and cared about all my life.

Memorial Sloan Kettering made me feel the horrors of cancer and the tortures of this kind of death.

Then I had to face Memorial myself. Was I about to face the same horrible fate or would I be one of the fortunate ones and cheat the grim reaper of death? Now six years later I have been struggling to keep going no matter what the pain or troubles. Dr. David Pfister, my oncologist, was the first to give me the name Lazarus, because he felt as though I kept coming back. I always tried to get Dr. Pfister to give me a number as to my statistical chance of survival, but he never would. His answer to my question was always the same, "Everyone has their own statistical number, which they hope is 100%."

However on one occasion, although he did not give me a number, he told me that there must be cancer in other places besides my neck because "how else did it get to your back?" I walked out of his office very depressed that day, but I decided not to let it get me. After all Lazarus made it and so would I.

On other occasions when the doctors were rather confused about my condition, I was called "an enigma wrapped up in a puzzle" by Dr. Mark Bilsky.

I suppose that Lazarus, too, confused the world.

2. ACCEPTING THE UNACCEPTABLE

My life has changed. I have gone from a self-assured successful executive with the world at my fingers, to someone far different. I spent years giving orders to my workers who did what I said partially because they believed it, and also to receive my recognition and acceptance. It has been an exciting life and I enjoyed it to the fullest extent possible.

But my philosophy about the importance of life has changed. I have been hit with the one of the biggest changers known to man. In the span of days, maybe hours, and finally minutes, one is transformed from a healthy, secure, successful individual with a life of certainty to a scared, insecure old man with the mention of just one dreaded word, cancer.

I sat in my favorite chair looking out over the Atlantic Ocean beating against the sandy beach one hundred feet below. It was my favorite chair in my favorite room, where I spent almost twenty winters enjoying my life of success and power. Life had been so great for my wife and I. We had our health and wealth, and a wonderful family that includes a stable of grandchildren. We roamed the earth through our travels, while I watched the business expand with great success.

Who would expect a little nodule on the side of my face to be anything other than a swollen gland? People get them all the time, but we decided to have it checked out just in case. When the doctor said he would make an appointment with a specialist to do a biopsy we were not too concerned. Although, it did seem a little upsetting that he made the appointment immediately.

Then the waiting began. Is there nothing as long as waiting for a lab result? Minutes feel likes days, and days like years.

There I sat when the telephone rang when my partner of a quarter of a century of good fortune, took the call in our bedroom. Those next ten or fifteen minutes felt much more like an eternity, than any I have ever spent. Finally, my wife came in and sat on the ottoman at my feet with her head resting on my thigh, I could feel the moisture of her tears on my skin. I needed no words.

From that moment on my life would no longer be the same. Seven years have gone by, and during that time I have become a very different person. The strong muscular man who walked miles each day with friends along the boardwalk had to learn to use crutches and a wheelchair. Pain became my unwelcome friend until morphine would come to my rescue.

The fourteen-inch rods put in my spine reduced my height by five inches. I had to overcome the terrible shock of my sudden reduction in height. Losing nearly a half-foot in height was an incredible blow to my ego. All of a sudden I was shorter than most of the people I knew. I would get up each morning and look at the picture of my wife and I that showed that I was taller than she, and try to remember those bygone days. Now I was at least three inches shorter than she. What was worse than the pain, and the blow to my ego, was my impaired ability to get places with ease.

I had to learn to live with this new self. This would be another task to achieve. I would have to learn to accept my new limitations. I would have to learn to take a dozen medicines a day; I would have to learn to apply pain-killing patches on my body every three days or relearn the ability to walk with crutches, wheel chair and eventually cane.

It was all almost too much to bear. But what were my alternatives? To take my life and give up all that I knew and loved? To become a vegetable and lay down on a couch with perennial self-pity or follow the philosophy shared by my cousin, Donald, who told me as he lay dying in Sloan Kettering Hospital, a line I shall never forget. Without remorse he said to me:

"These are the cards I was given, so these are the cards I must play."

There are some things in life about which we have no choice, so we must learn to accept them and play them the best way we can. So I learned to walk again, and look at life in a new way. I am going to live my life to the fullest extent accepting "the cards I was given to play, learning to accept pain, and keep going no matter what the price. I was going to use my every minute in the fullest way. I could learn to understand my limitations without regret, and use the experience to help others in a similar situation.

This I have done for seven exciting years even after I thought it was the end. I have climbed the volcanic rocks of Iceland with a brace and crutches and rode to the depths of the Egyptian Pyramids in a wheelchair. I have traveled around the world meeting new people, sharing my philosophy and experiencing new adventures that I may have never experienced otherwise. My bout with cancer has shown me the importance enjoying life the very best I can, and to accept my limitations with little regret, and with as much humor as I can muster. I have fought the battles of pain and depression and wounded ego along with Hamlet, Cyrano Du Bergerac, Don Quixote, Job, and my cousin Donald.

After a while, I took my experiences and began to share them with others. First over the Internet and most recently in a volume of stories published less than one year ago that is related to my travels despite my handicaps.

This is my belief: I have learned to accept the unacceptable. Learned to appreciate the trivial, and not to regret the regrettable.

I believe I have fought the battle of cancer the best way that I can, and have come through as well as I could.

3. THREE DAYS YOUNG—

Three Magical Minutes

This story is full of numbers, some torturous and others quite wonderful. It was tenth of May in 1997 and I was back from Florida for about sixty days. I was struggling with back pain for almost four months now. It had been a terrible time and even now, I hate to think of all the battles I fought in an attempt to overcome severe and constant pain. I had taken acupuncture for several weeks, and then I had fourteen applications of radiation. I was also taking different painkillers three or four times a day.

Finally I was admitted into Sloan Kettering, and I met with Dr. Mark Bilsky. He gave me the bad news that surgery would be necessary. He told me that the L-3 and L-4 lumbar section of my spine had basically disintegrated. After the surgery, I was in intensive care with a long recovery battle ahead. I would have to relearn the technique of walking, climbing up stairs and all the other ambulatory procedures we learn as kids. But for the moment, I was groggy and still recovering from the operation.

But across York Avenue there was excitement and relief. At last Sharon had her little baby girl! Her labor was slow in getting started, but one of my wonderful nurses, Kathy, gave Sharon some ideas about encouraging labor. Now Sharon was ready to go home to the west side of Manhattan with her little baby. Rachel was just three days old, as Sharon had stayed an extra day in the hospital, but was ready to start life on the other side of Manhattan. Sharon had not visited me since Rachel's birth because she was so very busy.

The Lying-in Hospital on 70th Street was not even three blocks from Sloan Kettering. As she left the hospital, Sharon thought about going home or walking the three short streets to visit me. She decided to risk it, although the hospital rules are strict about forbidding infants from visiting the intensive care area. I was half asleep and slowing coming back into the world of reality, when I suddenly saw Sharon walking toward my bed with a sweet little baby wrapped in swaddling robes.

Somehow Sharon must have known that I needed an incentive to recover because she laid little Rachel on my chest and in three minutes we bonded as with no one else. At that very moment, I knew I was determined to live to see little Rachel grow up. I remember she did not cry or even whimper although it was an unfamiliar environment. She lay passively on my chest, with what I like to think was a smile on her face, as I played with her little fingers. I was having a wonderful time and the pain just seemed to melt away. That little angel did more for me than all the treatments I was getting.

All of a sudden a jerky nurse came in and said, "What is SHE doing in here? Don't you know infants cannot visit the ICU (intensive care unit)?" Fortunately, not all nurses were like this one. As a matter of fact, most were sensitive and caring, and knew how much that interpersonal contact would mean to me over the next two months.

But it was too late, Sharon and baby Rachel had done their magic and no nurse however insensitive, could possibly undo those wonderful three minutes. Over the next two months, the repeated visits from so many family members and friends did help me to recover tremendously, but Sharon's visit with her little Rachel stands out in my mind as the turning point in my recovery.

4. THE WORST PART OF THE DAY

I am still drugged from the previous night's medicine. It is 1997 and I am experiencing my first of about one-half dozen hospital stays at Sloan Kettering Hospital. The lights come on at the ungodly hour of 5:00 A.M. as the night nurse finishes her eight-hour shift. She is no doubt thinking of going home, but as her day ends, my day in the hospital is about to begin once again. It has been four weeks now; four miserable, lousy weeks, with I.V.'s (Intravenous injections), MRIs, CAT scans, X-rays, and lord knows what else.

Every day begins with the same terrible routine. Since my operation, the stay at Sloan Kettering has been a drag like no other. The day begins with the night nurse taking my temperature and blood pressure. It never changes by more than a fraction; nevertheless they take it over and over again. It is now about 5:15 A.M. and I slept fitfully much of the night. Sometimes I could not be sure if I was awake or asleep. During the night I would hear noises, but I was not sure if I was hearing them or dreaming of them. I would always make a valiant attempt to go back to sleep, but the lights are really on, and another day was about to begin.

Then I hear a cheery new voice, "Good morning, Mr. W., I am going to be your day nurse today, my name is——. This is my first day on this floor. Let's get you washed up. Breakfast will be here in a few minutes."

It is now 5:30 A.M. Can you believe it?

Who cares what her name is, or whether she has been here before? I know that breakfast will not be there for another hour and one-half at the earliest, and when it comes the cereal will be cold and the scrambled eggs will be like shoe leather. I just want to go back to sleep. During the last four weeks I have shared the room with at least a half dozen patients. Most patients only stay for three or fours days after their operation. But I am a catch-22 patient. I needed to get infusions every twelve hours for my infection, but Medicare does not pay for such treatment at home. So even though it was costing approximately $3,000 a day to keep me in the hospital, already being paid by Medicare, they would not pay the $500 a day to treat me at home. You see, Medicare has regulations, and one of them is that they do not pay for drugs at home. So I remained in the hospital, while the insurance company, Medicare and Sloan Kettering fought over who would pay my drug bill, if I could in fact go home.

So weeks went by and I lived the daily routine of getting up at five in the morning, getting blood tests every six hours, having antibiotics fed intravenously twice a day and living the general annoyance of hospital life. It was like a never-ending nightmare.

Then, of course, there were the "rounds" every day, seven days a week for the past month. Sloan Kettering is a teaching hospital, so these young doctors would come in every morning as part of their education and part of my annoyance. Each day a group of doctors would come into my room and discuss my case with new interns and residents. One doctor would explain my case, and the students would ask the same questions. Sometimes I would say the answers before the doctor. There were the infectious disease interns, and the internal medicine students and the neurosurgical residents and any other team that may be around on a given day.

So the weeks dragged on and every day I would say to the various staff members who would listen, that it was costing another $3,000 for me to stay there today. The caring ones would respond sympathetically and say "Yes, we will get an answer soon." Others would just roll their eyes in frustration. "When will you get out of here? You will get out of here when you get out of here."

Finally, as the hospital bill approached $100,000 and after much discussion and bickering, my secondary insurance company agreed to pay the remaining drug bill and at long last I was on my way home.

5. THE TRAGEDY AT SLOAN KETTERING

In 1997 I was recovering slowly at Sloan Kettering. After the operation I was on the usual hook-ups with antibiotics, painkillers and Lord know what else. My life centered around my hospital room on the seventh floor and the hall where I did my physical therapy with Sammy and Justine. One day, Lila gave me the bad news that my cousin, Jerry's wife, Shirley, had been admitted to the eighth floor with head and neck cancer. I felt so badly for her knowing what she was going to go through.

One day after her operation I mustered the strength to visit her on the floor above. Jerry was staying with her and we had a short conversation to try to encourage each other. I tried to be optimistic, but I knew that she had a rough road ahead.

Jerry stayed by her bedside for days and nights on end. Once he came down to visit me and I could see what a toll this was having on him. He had already gone through a bout of cancer just a few years before. Then tragedy struck and not the way I had thought it would.

One evening Jerry left to go home to get a night's sleep.

The next morning as I awoke I heard two nurses talking. "It's his cousin. Someone should tell him."

I just knew that Shirley must have died during the night. But this was not yet to happen. When Jerry left the hospital at dusk the evening before, he walked across York Avenue to get his car.

As he crossed the street he was struck by a speeding car and apparently he was killed instantly. The car sped away and the hit-and run driver was never caught.

I was in shock as I was given the news. I could not believe it.

The family was devastated by Jerry's unexpected death, and then a short time later Shirley did die from her cancer. The uncertainties and tragedies of life are so terribly brutal. I think about how at that time I was uncertain about my prognosis, and then my cousin's accident proved again that we never know what the future holds for us or the reason for these events.

6. STRUGGLING WITH PAIN

Pain is insidious. It creeps up on you from all angles and in all forms and shapes. Some days I start out from my apartment pain—free and do not even think about it. I say to myself that today is going to be great, perfect for a nice trip to the museum, but then as I walk for one or two streets, it attacks my spine slowly and with cruelty. Then I realize that I did not even take my pain pills with me. Oh! What a stupid mistake, I think to myself. Suddenly, it dawns on me that I have not taken a pain pill in days. I do not even remember where my pills are.

I turn around and walk home slowly. When I get home I cannot find the pills. I had not had a pain pill in a day or two or maybe even three. My old pain is back to remind me of what it feels like once again. All of a sudden I start to feel shaky and tense. I go to the calendar and look at the date. Like a bolt of lightening I also realize that I am late with changing my pain patches. I rush to the box of duregisic fendynal, and cut open the patch box to put three new ones on my back and arms.

During the next twenty to thirty minutes, the morphine will gradually seep into my system from the surface of my skin. The pain begins to subside. The tension and anxiety begin to disappear. It always amazes me how fast three days seem to fly by. I must change those patches every three days like clock work or else I get terrible withdrawal symptoms. To get faster relief I look for and find my pill dispenser with the dilaudid pills and swallow a few.

The pain lingers from my lower back to the middle. I try to get in a comfortable position gradually and the pain subsides. I take a nap and after awhile I wake up and feel better. I thought about the six long years after my first spine operation, and my slow recovery at Sloan Kettering Cancer Center. After about ten weeks of radiation we flew back from Florida with the hope that maybe I was going to be better after all. Maybe I would actually be able to reschedule our trip to Antarctica.

I am basically an optimist, therefore I always think of the positive. This was one of those times. My back pains began four months before we had to cancel our trip to visit the last continent. After all, during those weeks of radiation what kept me going was the thought of getting to Antarctica.

After we got back to New York City from Florida the pain gradually subsided that spring. New York was warm and comfortable and I enjoyed walking its streets. But sadly, the pain gradually returned, and worst of all was it never seemed to subside. At that time, I was taking pain pills, but nothing as strong as morphine. Finally, I made an appointment with the neurosurgeon Dr. Mark Bilsky.

After taking a series of CAT scans and MRIs, Dr. Bilsky gave Lila and I the bad news about the disintegrated condition of the L3 and L4 lumbar section of my spine. I will never forget his description of the anticipated surgery. He described it as a battle, and he was the general. My back was the battlefield. The question he asked us out loud, but was really talking to himself was where would he attack? Should he go through the chest or the back?

I liked him from the start because he was a straight shooter. Dr. Bilsky said he wanted to wait a week to operate because he would like to have the "A" team. Much later I found out that this meant Dr. Bilsky wanted the spine surgeon, Dr. Borland, to be in the operating room. Dr. Borland was the best and my back needed the best.

Dr. Bilsky went on to describe that he would attack from the rear with the strategy of inserting rods into my back. These fourteen-inch rods were to be placed on either side of my spine to help support it, and would be attached with smaller pieces of hardware, much like one would buy at Home Depot.

This sounded simple enough, except when it would be done to my back. I am always reminded of a get-well card I once received from an old friend that questioned the difference between a major and a minor operation. Arnold's card answered the question. When it is mine, it is major. When it's yours, it is minor. There was no question mine was a major operation.

After the operation it was weeks before I could walk again.

The pain continued, but not quite as viciously, nevertheless it was present. After I had been in the hospital for weeks, Lila saw a notice for a lecture on pain that was to be given the next day. I went to the lecture hall in my wheelchair to listen to a nurse practitioner talk about the various approaches to pain management. One of the ways was the use of morphine patches. After the lecture I went up to the nurse practitioner and asked her if she would work with me. Nessa (Coyle) agreed and six years later, she is still working with me. She is a wonderful caring person and has always had time for me with her busy schedule.

Over the years Nessa has given me almost seventy-five prescriptions for fentanyl transdermal (through the skin) patches since I must get a new prescription every month. Sometimes I have taken as much as 400 micrograms or as little as 200 micrograms. Often people ask me how it feels to be taking morphine-based patches. My answer is always the same; "It is far better to be taking them, than not to be taking them. I would love to be a morphine addict for the next twenty years."

I must remember to change the patches every three days or else I suffer the consequences. I slowly develop a variety of symptoms from nausea to stomach cramps, to shakes or shivers. I am either freezing or sweating. When I begin to feel that way, I think I am getting ill, and even forget to attribute the symptoms to the patches. Typically, I will say to Lila, "I am getting sick, or I am catching the flu" or some such thing. Her first question is, "Did you change your patches?" My embarrassed answer is, "Oh, shit! I forgot!"

I maintain a schedule on my door and try to look at it every morning. The problem is when I forget. The concept is that the morphine patches gives you a certain level of pain relief and the dilaudid pills fill in when the pain gets greater, than the patches can control.

I see Dr. Tim Mahotra, the pain management specialist at Sloan Kettering about every six months. He prescribes patches and pills based on the level of pain that I have experienced. The concept of managing one's pain level is a rather recent one, and I would recommend it to anyone suffering from uncomfortable levels of constant pain. Dr. Tim's philosophy is why suffer from pain when you do not have to. I have learned that it is possible to suffer less with the help of these medications and lead a less painful life.

7. THE RACE WITH THE OVALTINE

After I got out of the hospital we tried to make life as normal as possible. One of our family routines was going to the supermarket. Each Friday we would go to Waldbaums to do our shopping for the week. When I first came out of the hospital I tried to use the walker while Lila pushed the food cart. I felt quite useless just hobbling around with not much to do. One day I noticed that Waldbaums had gotten in a new group of motorized carts for use by handicapped individuals. It was just the thing for me. I felt immediately comfortable as I got into the seat of one of the motorized carts. I turned on the motor and drove the cart up and down the aisles. At last I would be useful again and be able to reach over and put items into the cart's basket.

For two or three of the Friday shopping trips, I used the cart and it was just great. As a matter of fact I was feeling very productive once again. I became so comfortable I began to take a few chances, and found it was rather exciting.

One day I actually had a daydream about being in the Indy 500 of shopping cart races. In this dream NASCAR was the sponsor for a handicaps' race in shopping carts going around a track inside a huge supermarket designed for shopping carts. There were twenty of us racing around the aisles at brake neck speeds of eight miles an hour, around paper goods, into frozen foods, down the meat aisle, racing to the finish at fresh vegetables. I was neck and neck with some old lady whom I knew could not keep up with my amazing speed. I put my foot down to the floorboard and pushed my shopping cart to a dizzying speed of nine miles an hour, crossing the finish line in front of the checkout counter, one-half cart length before her. It was the highlight of my shopping cart racing career. What an incredible adventure! Would I ever become the Al Unser of shopping cart racing? Now I wondered if I could actually have such an experience.

Then one Friday evening the store was almost empty. I looked down an entire aisle and there was not a single customer loading merchandise into their cart. I thought to myself, wouldn't it be fun to get my shopping cart to somewhere near the nine miles an hour I had dreamed about? I put my foot down on the pedal as far as it would go and before I knew it, I was speeding past row after row of canned food, paper goods, and frozen foods.

I was having a great time. Because I was moving so fast, I did not notice that I came to the end of the cereals aisle. Then I suddenly realized that the aisle ended and I had to make a turn to keep from hitting the jellies right in front of me. So I made a quick right turn, which would not have been a problem, except for one fact. Directly in front of me was a pile of Ovaltine jars about five feet tall sticking out at the end of the next aisle. More quickly than one can say Ovaltine, I hit the pile head-on. Apparently they had not been installed very solidly because the jars seemed to fly out in every direction. I never though that there would be so many Ovaltine jars in one pile.

I recovered my composure, backed up and began moving away from the mess, just as a woman walked into the aisle. She reminded me of the old lady in my daydream who I beat out by a half cart length in our race. We stared at each other as I tried to smile. My quick wit came out with the following, "Isn't it a shame how sloppy they keep these stores nowadays?"

And I carefully drove away in my NASCAR shopping cart.

8. THE WHEELCHAIR ERA ENDS

A wheelchair is a rather intimidating implement as I found out during my several months sitting in one. Last month I finally returned my leased chair to the rental company. I no longer have it in my possession, so I can now write and talk about it frankly.

The truth is that getting mobility through a wheelchair is a terrible way to have to get around, except if you have no other choice. My experience began a few weeks after the series of operations on my back when the surgeons at Sloan Kettering put two 14" rods in my spine. After the surgery I spent weeks in the hospital relearning how to walk. It was an unbelievably difficult time.

First learning to stand, then using the walker with the help of the physical therapists and taking one little step at a time. I was so determined to do it that all my visitors would become my physical therapists. Of course all of my family members would come in, day after day to walk with me. My children Jack and Sabina would seem to be there almost all the time. Sometimes Sharon would sneak in with Rachel and Matthew because she lived so close by. Then there were, my friends, Joel and Barbara, for example, who became two of my favorite helpers. They did not put any extra pressure on me to learn to walk faster. They seemed to be very casual about it. For example, Joel would tell me about all the problems they were having in the new company in San Jose as he walked along side me.

I remember the most difficult task to conquer was learning how to walk upstairs and downstairs. I had a terrible fear of falling backwards as I attempted to take the first step. I was extremely unsteady on my feet for weeks after the operation, so I worried that I would fall down the steps. The first time I tried a step I needed two physical therapists to be at my side. There was Justine beside me and Sammy behind me. They were wonderfully patient with this patient. Gradually I overcame my fear and after a while I started to think about going home. Of course, it was one thing was to go home, and another thing to get around the neighborhood. That was where the wheel chair came in. I had an aide for a few hours a day and she would take me downstairs to get around the town.

No matter how my physical condition was, I had to be a traveler even to get around the Upper East Side of Manhattan.

That was where the aide and the wheel chair came in. First we would go to the end of the street and watch the boats pass by on the East River. Then we would go the local park on East 76 Street and watch the kids playing in the park. I would often go with Sharon, Matthew and Rachel. They would race around the park and I would sit in the wheel chair thinking how great it would be to be able to run around with them. I would also think to myself, was I ever going to be able to play with them again? Then it was on to Central Park. Sharon and Jeff had moved to 100th Street and Central Park West. There were parks all around the place.

As I write about it, I pray with all my might that I will never have to use a wheelchair again. Here are some of the difficult issues.

The first unpleasantness was the height that it puts one at.

You are from one to two feet below the rest of the world. I remember going to a parade along Fifth Avenue one day that was an absolutely discouraging experience. About all I could see were coats and jackets of everyone in front of me. Every once in a while we would find a considerate group of folks that would let us get in front, but most of the time it was very difficult to maneuver the wheelchair in a crowd.

Another unpleasant experience was that almost any conversation was held with your pusher and not you. If we stopped to have a conversation with someone, the person would address his or her words to the person standing behind me and not to me. It was as though I was mentally, as well as physically on a lower level. It was not that I was treated with disrespect, but I felt ignored unintentionally in conversation, as the person seemed to look over me and in the direction of the person pushing my chair. Even if I asked the question, the answer would be directed at the person behind me.

Lastly, sitting in a wheelchair is like being on a rocky road to everywhere. You seemed to notice every little crack in the sidewalks of the streets of the City of New York. Fortunately, many of the sidewalks in the city have ramps on the corners, but when you reach a corner that does not have one, it is an uncomfortable maneuver to get across. Your helper turns you about, then tips you back you feel as though you are falling out of the thing.

But now at last, or at least I hope it is the last, all of that is behind me. The wheel chair has been returned the Medical Supply Company and my adventures in the wheelchair are at an end.

9. National Cancer Survivor's Day

I received a flier from the Suffolk Y announcing that next Wednesday was National Cancer Survivors Day. There was going to be a panel of speakers who were all cancer survivors. They were going to speak about the different ways they have coped with the disease. The bottom of the flier invited others in the public who wanted to could speak on ways they have coped with the disease.

In just a few weeks I would be off to France, but thought it might be a good idea if I could join the group. I called the chairperson the next day and was told that they already had a panel of eight, but at the end of the session there would be a period of time for comments where I would be able to speak for a few minutes.

When I arrived there were about forty people, mostly women in the audience. The leader announced that each speaker was a breast cancer survivor and started out by saying

"I have survived cancer for (blank) years."

As each woman stood up, she stated the number of years that she had survived.

It sounded as if they were members of Alcoholics Anonymous. All of them were enthusiastic and that was probably the most important fact of all. Each speaker spent a few minutes telling her struggle and the program that helped her to survive. Several women said diet was their salvation, and some gave the diets that helped them most. Another woman told of the exercise program she developed. She asked the people in the audience to stand and join her in doing several exercises. She then invited survivors to join her exercise group held weekly at the Y. Still another woman told of her Tai Chi program and gave a demonstration.

It was exciting to hear how each found her method to fight the disease. Then, the chairwoman invited speakers from the audience. Two or three went before I raised my hand to speak.

I started out by stating that I was first diagnosed with cancer in the winter 1995. I told them about my operations, radiation treatments, and how I asked Dr. Eliot Strong, Head and Neck surgeon at Sloan Kettering Hospital, if I could travel again.

I then read the statement from the back cover of my new book, <u>The Chinese Walking Stick</u>, quoting Dr. Strong who said, "travel does not affect the growth of cancer cells." I will never forget how he told me to use my time the best way I could. Then, I told the audience how I have taken his words to heart, and have traveled all over the world since.

I told the audience how this philosophy has worked for me. I concluded by saying not to concern yourself with the amount of inheritance money left for your children, but to enjoy the excitement of seeing the world.

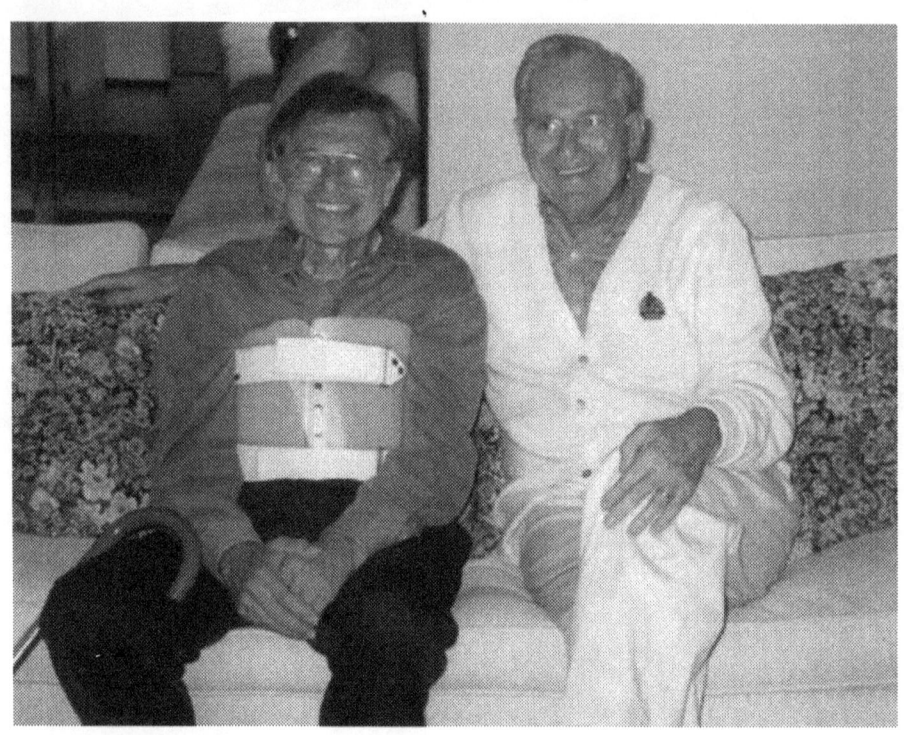

Gene and Jim After Retirement

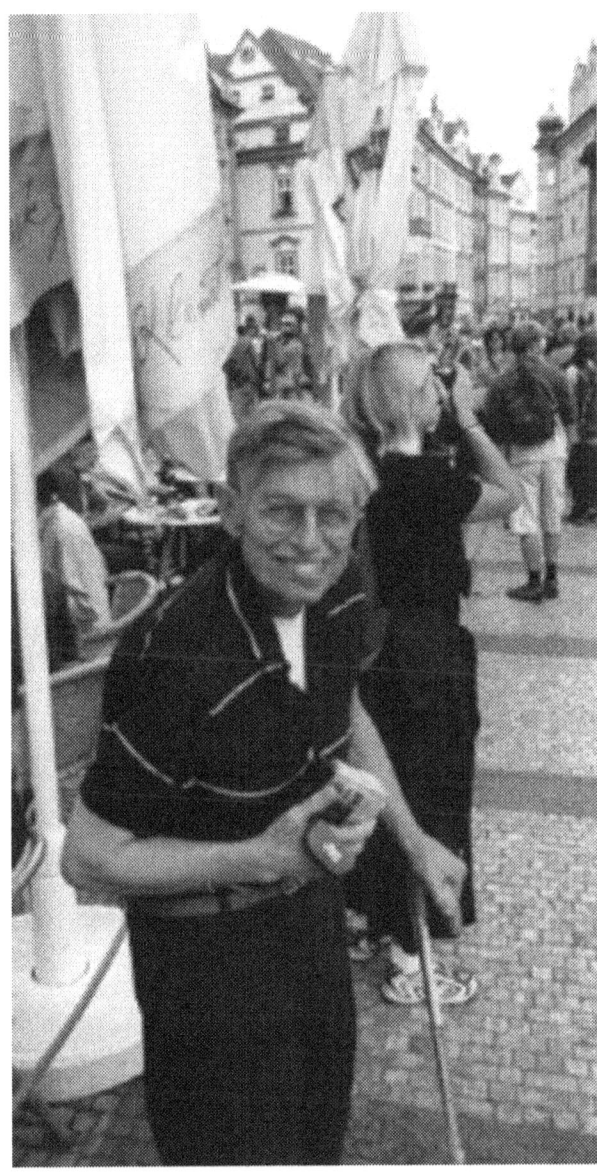

Visiting Prague

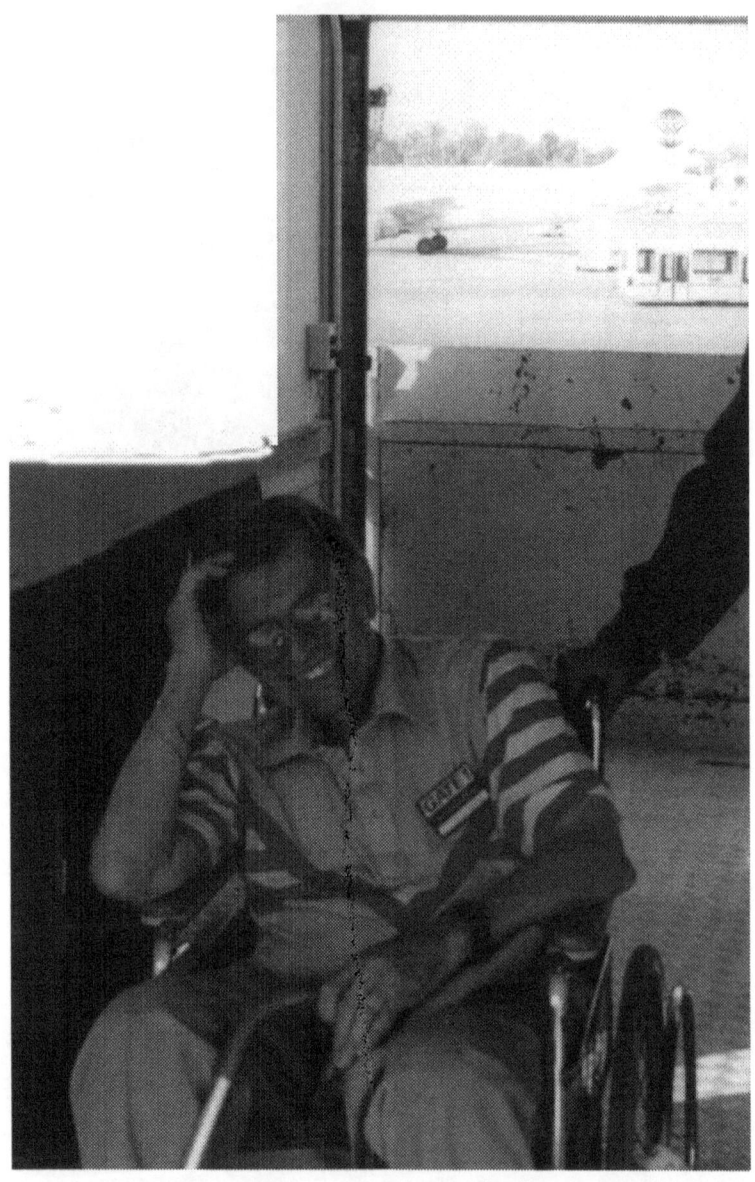

The Wheelchair Era

Chapter Five: Kiddie Tales

Dedicated to the Family: Children and Grandchildren

1. KISS CASSANDRA

Occasionally my family likes to have a family sleepover in our apartment in Manhattan. It is a beautiful place three hundred and fifty feet above the streets of New York. We have a magnificent view of the East River crossed by a half dozen emblazoned bridges. The kids love to stand on the window ledge and watch the tankers sail under the bridges. Every once in awhile, one child will scream out, "Look at that helicopter!" or "Here comes another ship!" Typically, everyone strains to find the mentioned object outside of the window. After a while they discover a new object and everyone runs in that direction.

As the sun begins to set and the city lights come on, the New York skyline becomes a mass of light flooding from scores of skyscrapers. Sometimes we all sit down to play one card game or another. All of us from age six to seventy-six have a great time. After the games are over, desserts and cookies are served, and the ritual of reading stories to one another begins. Every single child, parent and grandparent has a marvelous time.

As the evening progresses, it becomes apparent that the children will soon be ready for bed. But in our apartment there are not enough beds for all, so the routine has been for the kids to sleep on the living room floor, large enough for all. The living room is laid out with sheets, pillows, and blankets in a line for all the tired kids.

During one particular sleepover, we had extra guests in addition to the grandchildren. There were Sharon's children, Matthew and Rachel and Marc's three children, Elizabeth, Daniel, and Abigail. Elizabeth and Daniel brought two of their best friends. Elizabeth invited Christina, and Daniel invited Christina's younger sister Cassandra. Since Elizabeth is older than the rest, she was not yet ready for sleep.

Everyone else was careful to arrange his or her sleeping arrangements by gender. Daniel and Matthew had bunks closest to the archway, while Abigail, Rachel and Cassandra were side by side.

When the children were comfortably bedded down in their locations, each of the adults went down the line to kiss each child good night. I was the last adult to take the journey and started with Daniel, then Matthew, Abigail and Rachel.

As I bent down to give Rachel a kiss, I suddenly realized that she was looking at Cassandra who was right next to her. I was not sensitive enough to pick this up. When I began to move away because I had not planned to kiss Cassandra, I suddenly felt a tug on my shirtsleeve. I turned back to see Rachel looking at Cassandra and then, looking toward me. Rachel sensed that Cassandra was expecting a kiss, and was about to be disappointed by not getting one.

Then, in her quiet way, Rachel pulled my head down to her face and whispered in my ear, "*Kiss* Cassandra, Papa." I did as she suggested. When I bent down and kissed that very sweet girl on the cheek, Cassandra gave me the happiest smile. And we were both oh, so delighted. I looked over to Rachel, my sensitive little granddaughter and went back to give her another kiss.

The smiles on their faces told me just how happy they were that I did that. Rachel was able to read her little friend's expression so well that she knew a kiss is what Cassandra also wanted. Rachel has that special talent of looking into one's eyes and reading their feelings. I have always wished that I could do that as well. Within minutes all of those tired little kids were fast asleep.

As I look back over days gone by, and try to think of happy times, the few minutes shared with those two little girls stands out as a very special experience.

2. MOM AND POP PENGUIN

Parenthood is quite an obligation. Our species has found that it is a very difficult task to raise kids; to teach them right from wrong; not to drink and not to smoke; to hang out with the right crowd; and to know the importance of a good education. We often have to sacrifice a lot to bring them up in the way we would like them to be.

But on the opposite end of the world, there is a species that probably sacrifices a lot more than we do. They work harder to have their offspring, than any other species I have ever studied. I am most impressed with the way the Empress Penguins sacrifice to keep their species from disappearing from the face of the earth.

First, the female lays her single egg, which takes a lot out of her. She then immediately returns to the sea and stays there for almost four months to gain strength and nourishment. In the meantime, the male must stand over the egg for the next four bitterly cold months, waiting for his mate to return. From what I understand the most difficult time for any species to endure is the period of protecting its eggs while they wait for them to hatch. They must endure hurricanes, minus 80-degree freezing weather, and continuous sixty mile an hour gales.

The Empress Penguin must stand over his eggs in an upright position to keep them warm in these intolerable conditions. Now keep in mind that during those four months they are not getting any nourishment. During all this time they are only living off their own body fat. By the time their mate returns from the sea, the male has lost about fifty percent of his body weight. What an incredible sacrifice for that little guy who is about to hatch, the penguin might think.

In the meantime, the female must survive the rigors of the ocean. This is not living at the Club Med. She must find food and strengthen herself for her swim back home to her mate. She must constantly be on alert to avoid becoming food for the sea lions or the elephant seals. If for some tragic reason she does not make it back, her mate will stand over his egg, until he has no further energy left. Sadly enough sometimes he must abandon the egg and leave it to die as he swims back out to sea.

One of the characteristics I understand is that penguins, like humans, have a sense of humor. I imagine that when the female penguin makes it back and somehow or other miraculously finds the right mate, she waddles up to him and says,

"Irving, Are you all right?"

"Molly, just where have you been?" asks Irving.

"Moisha is about to hatch and you have been gone too long.

What kind of mother are you going to be anyway? I'll bet you have been shopping at Bloomies' boutique for the past few months. Yetta and Sarah came back three days ago."

"All right, all right already, Irving. I just stopped off for a herring snack at Katz's. I needed some energy. You know I am not as young as I used to be. And you know I needed a new formal gown for the bris."

"Okay, okay." says Irving. "It's your turn to take over, Moisha has been kicking up a storm for the last two weeks. I am going for a swim. I'll see you in a couple of months."

I have often wondered how many humans would be able to be parents if they had to stand over a five pound eight ounce baby for a few months? Can you picture how a mother would survive if she had to do that? Think of the sacrifices parent penguins have to make. Perhaps parents of human babies should take a lesson in "penguin upbringing" before they have their own children. Well, maybe it would not be a good idea, on second thought, there would probably be far less children born to humans.

3. Matthew & Me on a Bus

Manhattan is a city of pocket parks. There must be one hundred of them scattered throughout Manhattan Island alone. Recently I called my daughter and said that I needed a "grandchild fix". I had been away for ten days on a rainy vacation and when I came back, I felt like playing with Matthew and Rachel my four and two year old grandchildren who live on the Upper West Side of Manhattan. Sharon said that she was going to her old neighborhood around the 70's and Amsterdam Avenue to visit a playground. I said, "How would you like company there?" and Sharon said, "Sure. We will be there at twelve."

I already felt good upon my 12:30 P.M. arrival when I saw three smiling faces in three peak caps. I sat with Sharon watching Matthew and Rachel run around the playground, up the slides, down the slides, around the climbing poles, on the elephants, and off the donkeys. I took pictures both with and without the peak caps. While Sharon and I talked every once in awhile, they would race over and give me a fast hello and a kiss.

Sharon commented, "They missed you."

"I missed them too." I said.

After about an hour Rachel started to drag. She slowed down to a crawl and I could see she was really tired. Now when she came over to say "hello" she walked over more slowly, put her head in Sharon's lap. At this point Sharon said, "She's ready for a nap."

Matthew was at the other end of the playground having a great time with some new friends. I said to Sharon, "How about if I stay with Matthew here at the playground and you take Rachel home for her nap."

She said, "Would you? I think he would love that."

"Sure." I said. "I can take him home on the bus."

Matthew overheard that he was staying in the playground with Papa. He thought it over for a split second and said, "OK." Then ran back to play on the monkey bars.

As Sharon left with Rachel, she said, "Are you sure you can handle Matthew in the bus with the cane and all?"

"Oh sure" I said, "No problem."

Matthew played with his new friends John, age two and Gracie, age four, while I talked with their mother. After a while little John started to get cranky and his mother said that he needed to go home and take a nap. But unlike Rachel, John did not want to go home. He just cried and got more upset. Finally their mother said, "let's go for ice cream!" This was a great way to separate them from the park. Off they went in their two-child carriage.

A minute later Matthew said, "Can I go for ice cream?"

We had been there quite a while and I also thought it was about time to leave.

I said, "Sure. What kind do you like?"

"Chocolate." was his instant reply.

We walked out of the playground, hand in hand. In my left hand I had my cane and in my right was my four-year old pal, Matthew.

We stopped off at the 77th Street ice cream and yogurt bar. We each ordered a chocolate kiddy cone. The teenage girl serving ice cream was quite generous with her portions, so we each walked out with a big cone topped with colorful sprinkles on a large scoop of double chocolate ice cream. As an after thought I went back and grabbed a handful of paper napkins, just in case the ice cream started dripping.

We stood outside the store enjoying the sprinkles and ice cream for several minutes. We did not talk, as we were too busy relishing our treat. In time we gradually started walking to the bus stop only about a block away. I hooked the cane on my left arm, so that I could continue licking my ice cream and also hold Matthew with my right hand. We got to the bus stop with no problem, each of us licking away.

It was delicious, but as it always happens with ice cream, eventually they started to melt. This fact did not stop either of us. I looked at Matthew and suddenly realized that his face was pretty much covered with ice cream, as was his right hand up to his wrist. He was enjoying it too much to miss a lick though, but did not seem to like the feeling of ice cream on his hands. I used several napkins on his sticky fingers. I realized that he had some on his jacket as well. I used some more wiping around his pocket. I used the last two napkins to wrap around the cone because the original one given to us by the server was completely doused in chocolate.

It was at this time that Matthew says, "Papa, you hold it." My right hand positioned Matthew's cone at mouth level for him to continue licking away in ecstasy, while I continued to lick my own cone. We just stood at the bus stop enjoying ourselves. Even allowing three buses pass by. While I was too busy to even think about getting on, Matthew who is very bright noticed and said, "Isn't that our bus?"

I said," OK we will take the next one." Then at that same moment a bus stopped right in front of where we stood. It was too convenient to let it go, so we climbed onto the bus. I am not sure just how we made it, though. My left hand held two ice cream cones with my cane hooked on the elbow, while my right hand held Matthew's hand, and I had my bus pass in my mouth. Somehow I was able to manipulate the bus pass into the machine and get it out again.

That was a complete success. I looked over at Matthew who never missed a lick of his ice cream. I maneuvered Matthew so that we could stand by a pole. Nobody got up to give us a seat since the whole front section of the bus was filled with a brigade of white-haired women. But actually, Matthew and I were doing fine except for the dripping Ice cream. Finally one nice old lady searched in her pocket book and found about a dozen tissues. By this time it was a lifesaver because I was completely out of napkins. I used two of them to rewrap Matthew's cone, and two of them for my cone, which was also dripping a lot.

Finally a woman said that she was getting off at the next stop, I think it was 86th Street. Matthew hopped into the seat and I squeezed in next to him; he pulled my arm to his mouth to finish licking his ice cream. Luckily, I had finished mine by then. My major task was to keep the ice cream from dripping all over Matthew's jacket. His face was completely covered with ice cream, so I used the last few tissues to wipe his nose, cheeks and chin. No possibility of wiping his mouth because he was too busy licking. At last Matthew finished his cone.

When I had finally managed to wipe the last bit of ice cream from Matthew's face, the woman next to me says, "Pardon me, I am getting off at this stop." I swung my legs out, so she could get around me, but upon a second look I realized that she must weigh 250 pounds and could not possibly get by without my getting up. Somehow I held the cane, juggled the dirty napkins and steered Matthew to stand, while getting up myself.

As she finally raised her massive body she screamed just as the bus was about to leave her stop, "I am getting off HERE." The bus driver reopened the door, and this woman gave me one last dirty look, and waddled off.

We had just reseated when I looked out the window and realized that our stop was next. I dropped the wad of tissues on the seat and made our way to the exit.

We were in great shape as we walked toward Central Park West and passed a big firehouse on our left.

Matthew says, "Papa, let's see the pole!"

"What did you say?" I did not understand his sentence.

"You know, what they have in the firehouse."

"Oh! You mean the fireman's pole. Where they slide down to get into the engines?

"Yeah" he said, "Let's see it!"

"Matthew, I am a little tired right now. Let's go some other day."

4. PAPA, PAPA, IT IS A SING-ALONG

"Papa, Papa, Papa." A soft hand pressed my arm as I gradually arose from a deep sleep. It was about eight o'clock in the morning on the last Friday before Christmas. I opened my eyes to see Rachel and Sharon standing at my bedside saying something. Eventually I began to understand what they were asking me.

Rachel said, "Can you come to school this morning to hear the Christmas sing-along?" When the words come from Rachel, for me most always the answer, is "yes."

Sharon began to fill in all the details. "At ten o'clock there is a sing-along in the school auditorium. Rachel would like you to come. She also would like it if you could video it."

"Oh!" I said, "I don't know if I have the camera here."

"If you don't have one, Sharon said, "I can always get it from another family."

I got up from bed without any knowledge of the time. But Sharon said, "You do not have to get up now, you can sleep for a while."

Rachel said, "But you have to get there early because it is so hard to park."

As they left my room to get the bus, I said, "Oh, I'll get there in plenty of time." I laid back to sleep for a few more minutes…

…Until I heard my grandson Daniel playing the piano loudly. I woke up startled without any idea what time it might be. I reached for the television remote and pressed the 'ON' button. The CNBC station flashes 10:13 E.S.T. as the time. Even in my half-stupor, I know E.S.T. means Eastern Standard Time, and not the time somewhere else such as Chicago or California.

I flew out of bed, grabbed my pants and ran to the bathroom to finish dressing, while I looked for my cane and keys. As I rushed to turn the TV off, I noticed the time is now 10:17 A.M. not even five minutes since I woke with a jumpstart, but a "commitment is a commitment." Then I remembered I told little Rachel that I would be there by ten and here it was, way past ten and I was not yet out the door.

I opened the garage door and turn on the engine only to find that Marc parked his car directly behind mine.

"Marc!" I yell. "Move your car!"

"Can you wait five minutes?" Marc asked.

"I am just eating my cereal and my shoes aren't on."

"Five minutes is too long, when you are a half hour late!" I shouted, "Throw me your keys!"

I got into his rental car, but could not find the emergency brakes, so I drove with them on and got the car on the street in one piece. I jumped into my car and turn out of our block, headed for the school. I look at the clock it is 10:19 A.M. and I comically thought of "the Diller, the Dollar and the ten o'clock" rule. I could not believe that only seven minutes have passed since I rolled out of bed.

I arrive at the school at 10:23 A.M. and of course, Rachel was quite right about the streets around the school being jammed. There was not a parking space in sight. I rolled right up to the school, and took a chance by parking next to the entrance where a sign reads "No parking: Fire Zone." I race out of the car and into the building and ask the first person I see for the auditorium. She says, "Take a left at the next aisle, listen for the din and you will see a dozens or so parents still trying to get in.

I followed her directions and reached the door. The auditorium must have had one thousand or so parents and children sitting on the floor, but I squeezed and I pushed and finally got in.

Hundreds of children were sitting up tall and all were looking straight ahead, with the exception of one little girl. Oh, what a thrill! I went wild when I spotted my little grandchild who was waving and giving me a wonderful smile. I was certain that Rachel was looking for me. But then I got another big thrill! Because I spotted my grandson Matthew among the older students.

This sing-along day was a wonderful time for me to share with my grandchildren. I am so happy that I got up in the nick of time.

5. Katie and the Chicks or Tora, Tora, Tora

My cousin Joe and I arrived in Salacroup, France after a long two-hour ride from the city of Rodez. I was tired from the past two weeks of touring and looked forward to being settled at Robert and Carol's house for a one-week stay. Although Joe, Robert and Carol were friends for a decade or more, this was my first introduction to them, and I was still given a warm welcome, as if we were old friends.

It was so generous of them to give me a room for one week. I wanted them to feel as though I would be a good guest, but I was so tired that it was impossible for me to be very sociable. I was invited to my room almost as soon as we arrived. They even went to the trouble of putting up mosquito netting, so I would not be uncomfortable during the night. I was asleep the instant my head hit the pillows.

The next morning we were up bright and early, ready to be introduced to the little town of Salacroup. When I came out of the backdoor, Robert and Joe were already working in the vegetable garden. I fell in love with the place in an instant. The house is on a few acres of beautiful rolling hills with a babbling brook at the end of their property. I walked around from one end to the other breathing in the fresh air of southern France. By the time I walked back to the vegetable garden, I felt completely at home.

Out of the corner of my eye, I saw Katie racing over to say hello. Although I met Katie the previous evening, I was now ready to make friends. As soon as she saw me, she came running over with Nora, the gray and white chick, tucked under her arm. When she reached me, Katie warmly shoved Nora into my arms, and said, "This is Nora!" I held the little chick carefully because she was so light that I felt I could crush her with one extra squeeze.

Katie was a bright nine year old who loved to read books. She had an expressive smile with bright blue eyes and had long, light-brown hair that flowed casually over her face. As soon as I saw her she reminded me of my granddaughter Rachel. Katie was such a fast talker that I had to listen intensely to keep up.

A minute later she raced off in the direction of the cage. In an instant she was back with Tora, the redheaded chick, and not wanting to show any bias, Katie grabbed Nora away from me and gave me Tora instead. However, Tora was very shy, and reluctant to be held. The next thing I knew Tora flew to the top of my head and stayed there just as motionless as I. Sensing our discomfort, Katie grabbed Tora from my head, and raced off with Nora and Tora under each arm.

My initial meeting with Nora and Tora was over. I hoped I made a good impression, but I was not sure. Katie put both chicks back into the cage and raced over to help Joe plant the lettuce. I went in to have breakfast.

I thought what a wonderful little girl. I hoped that she liked me as much as I liked her. She was a girl full of excitement, which I could believe had the philosophy, "Why walk when you can run?" She ran everywhere with a great spirit and full of energy.

In the afternoon, I helped Robert, Joe, and Katie with the vegetable garden. The ground was very hard, so it took a lot of effort just to break up the soil. Katie used some of that boundless energy to break up the rock-solid earth. I tried the best I could to help, but it was not easy to balance a shovel and a cane simultaneously. No one complained about my contribution, so I presume I did not inhibit their progress too much.

That evening we all went out to a restaurant for dinner. We had a very nice French dinner, despite Katie's reluctance to going out to eat. As soon as we came home, Katie went into the chicken coop to check on the chicks. When she returned it was obvious that she was distressed.

Katie found the gray and white chick, Nora, in the coop, but Tora, the flaming redheaded chick was nowhere in sight. We all looked for her to no avail. We searched in the shed and in the basement. We looked in the fields and in the vegetable garden. Tora was nowhere to be found. The next morning we continued the search. We looked all over Salacroup, which consists of ten or so houses and an equal number of barns and sheds.

Then Robert saw a neighbor's dog sneaking around the cellar door and by the look on its face, Robert felt sure that the dog had somehow gotten into the chicken coop and made off with Tora.

Katie was quietly broken hearted. She walked around holding Nora, but all the time called for Tora. All over the little town she searched for her missing chick. Up and down one street, and then to the end of the other, as she called her little friend. I could hear her plaintiff voice in the distance, "Tora, Tora, Tora."

Wherever Katie went she brought Nora with her. I thought it was a pity for this little girl to experience sadness so early in life, but that is part of life's journey. Fortunately for Katie, she had her little friend Nora to keep her company and soon Nora became part of the family. She ate with the family and slept with the family. When Carol would read Katie a story in the evening before bedtime, the little chick sat right next to Katie. She was definitely a full member of the family.

Meanwhile, it was time to return to the United States. Joe and I said goodbye to Robert, Carol, Katie, and of course, I gave Nora a good-bye kiss after Katie put her on my shoulder. Joe also gave the chick a good-bye kiss.

I recently heard from Robert who informed me that since the family returned to California, he found a local farmer in the Salacroup area who became Nora's caretaker for the winter. The update is that in the last few months, Nora has grown into a larger hen and is doing fine while waiting for Katie to return to France next summer to see her pal.

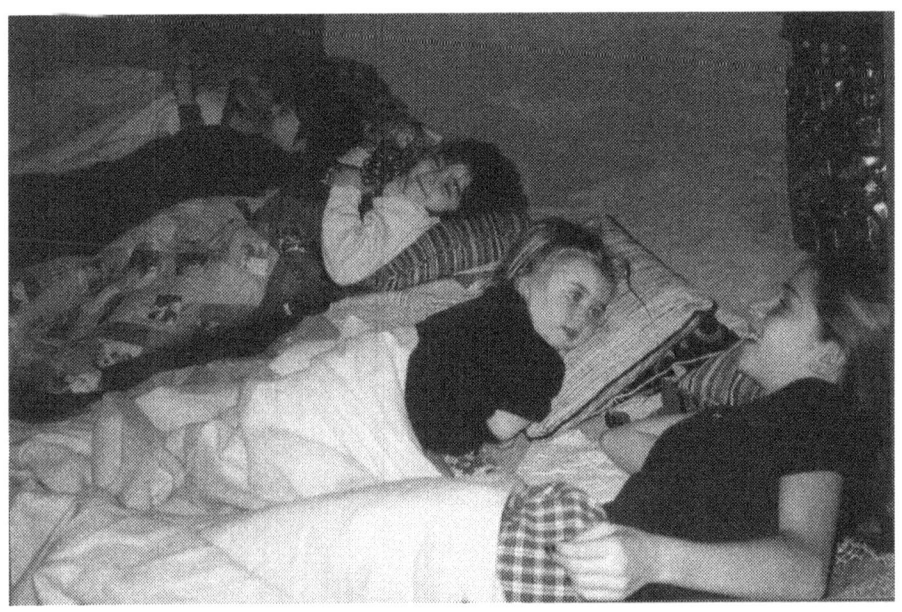

Kiss Cassandra

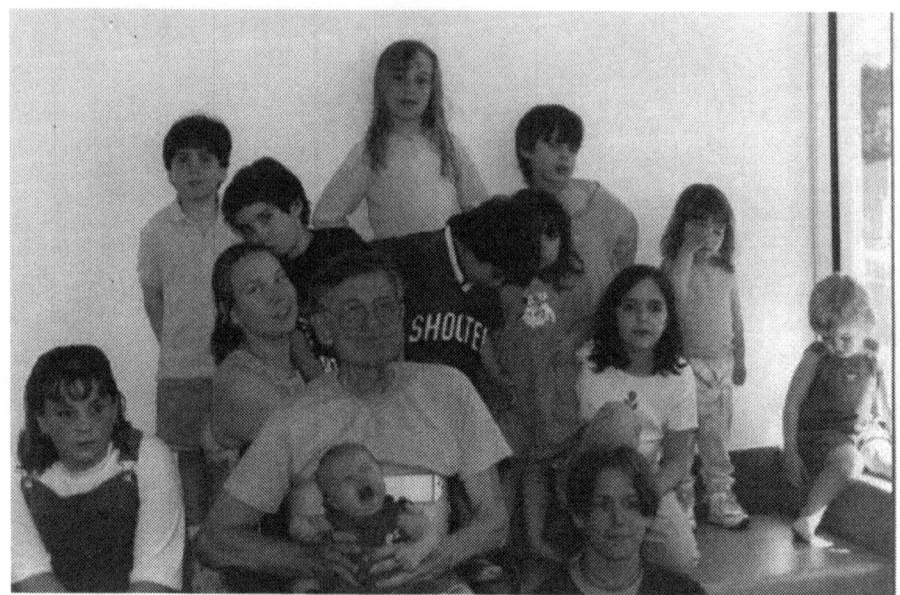

Gene and the Grandchildren

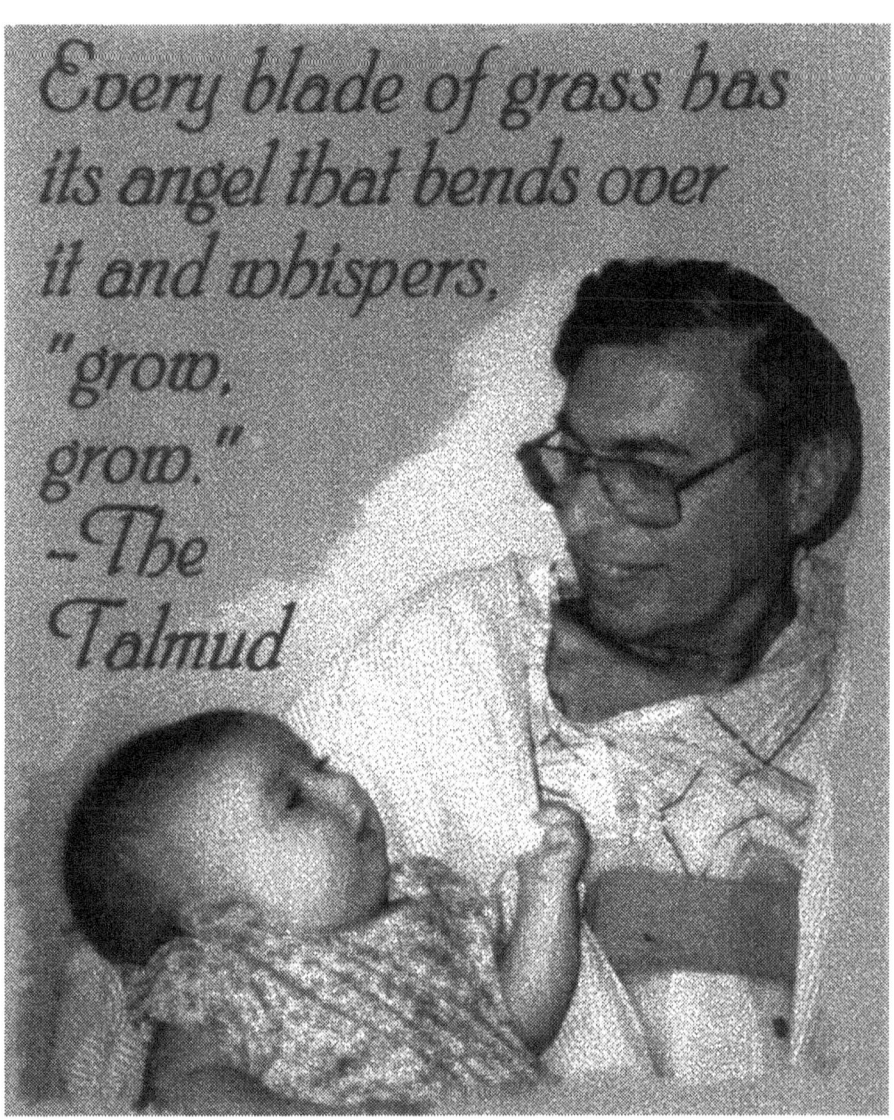

Grow, Grow, Grow!

Chapter Six: Local Tales

Dedicated to Our Great City

1. FARE'Y TALES OF OLD NEW YORK

My Grandmother, Julia Holstein and Grandfather, Isaac Sprung were life-long New Yorkers. They married in the 1870's in the lower East Side of the city having come from Europe as teenagers. He was a furrier and she worked in a factory as a milliner. They were a very prolific pair having twelve children over a span of twenty or so years.

She was a hardworking lady and very successful manager of a household. After arriving in the city, they lived their entire life in various corners of New York City, initially on the lower East Side, then moving to Harlem, and finally to the suburbs of Rockaway. They were one of the first families to have automobiles. But before acquired that very modern means of transportation, their method of travel in our very busy and crowded city was by trolley car. Electric power driven trolleys were the most popular way of getting around the city in the latter half of the nineteenth century The cost of each trip was the very economical cost of one nickel.

In the winters I can imagine my grandmother, a stout woman not over five feet tall, running around the city dressed in her fur coat, made naturally in my grandfather's fur shop. In those days augmenting the coat, she would have on a fur muff to keep her hands warm.

In my mind, I can see her laden down with packages getting on the trolley and searching for her nickel to put in the slot. It was a daunting task especially when she would sometimes be accompanied by a few of her one dozen kids.

She would come home to her household and make dinner for a family of so many. When Grandpa would get home after a hard day cutting furs, he would hear her complaints of her day in the city.

Then she would end the talk by saying how hard it was to get the nickel out to put it in the trolley slot. After listening to her complaints for half the winter, he said, "I have an idea. I am going to put that little purse in the muff so you will just be able to put your hand in and get the coin out."

"Oh! yeah! You said that before. All talk. So do it already!"

But this time he came through. A few nights later he came home with package wrapped in the Daily Forward, announcing, "Here is your present, Julia." She had forgotten all about her complaint by then. She opened it up and to her surprise was a beautiful new muff with a clip in the center and underneath it was the little purse just big enough to put in several coins. It was a wonderful idea and she put it on, right at the dining room table. It felt warm and comfortable and oh so practical. In a minute she mastered the idea of unbuttoning the purse, getting the coin out without fishing through her pocket book, which was still at her elbow. She went over, kissed Isaac and then cleared away the dinner dishes.

The next afternoon Julie went shopping with her brand new muff. As she boarded the trolley, she put her hand inside the purse and pulled out her nickel as if by magic from the center of the muff. Soon crowd of ladies all wanted to know why she did not have to fish through her pocketbook. She showed them her new muff with the purse hidden inside. Julia became the talk of the town and the Sprungs sold their new muffs to fur shops all over the city.

Of course the idea could have been copied except for one fact. A few days before Isaac, who had become knowledgeable about the ways of American society went down to the United States Patent office and asked for an application. Before long a letter arrived in the mail from the Patent Office and Isaac celebrated the receipt of their first Sprung patent, Number 526,950. Grandpa brought home a bottle of Champaign and made a toast to Grandma's warm hands.

For the next thirty years or so as the tale goes, the ladies of New York were able to take their nickels out of their muff on cold winter days to comfortably pay their fare when they climbed aboard the trolleys.

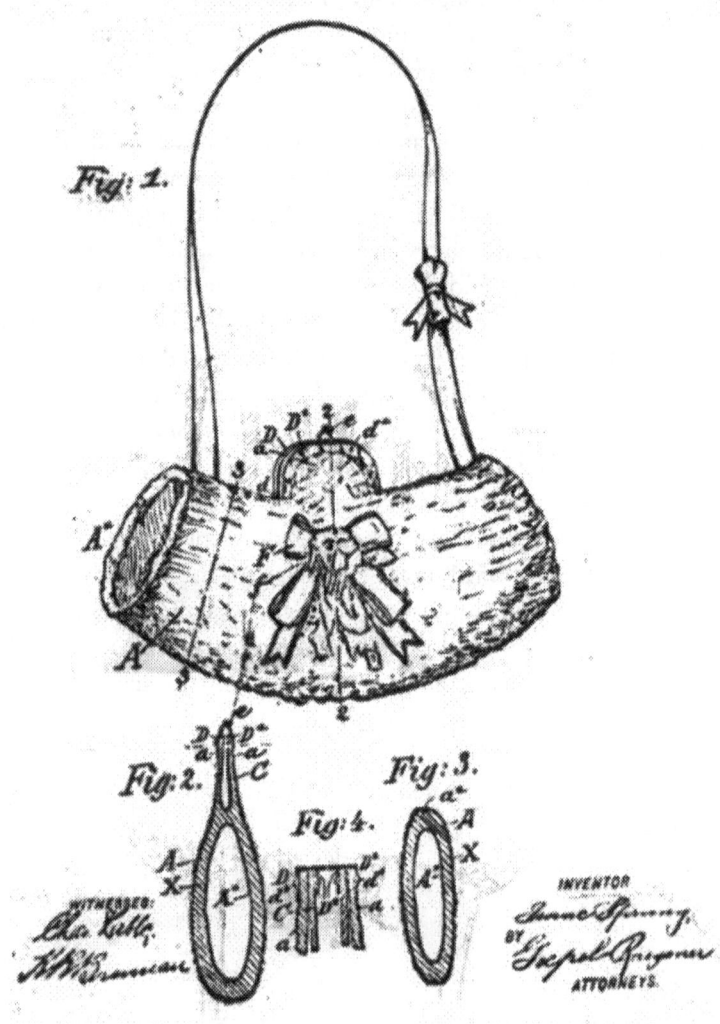

(No Model.)

I. SPRUNG.
COMBINED MUFF AND PURSE.

No. 528,960.   Patented Oct. 2, 1894.

U.S. Patent for Muff and Purse

2. GOING, GOING, GONE

One of my favorite daytime occupations since I retired is going to Sotheby's to see all the wonderful items going up for auction. From Persian oriental carpets to impressionistic paintings from all over Europe, Sotheby's would have them on auction. It was such fun to walk through their aisles and see what next great works of art were going to be sold to the highest bidder.

I have often said that going through Sotheby's is better than visiting the Metropolitan Museum of Art. They have great works of art, right on my corner, not often crowded and free to view. What more can I ask? Naturally, a story to write as you will find out.

One October day I noticed that Sotheby's was advertising a photographic exhibit. On the cover of the brochure was a picture of a factory by Alfred Stieglitz. The day before the actual auction I walked through the wonderful exhibition of those black and white pictures of the forties and fifties.

I thought it would be quite an experience to see the actual auction. So the next day with nothing to do, I decided to sit in on the auction. I arrived just a few minutes before 2:00 P.M. The main auction gallery was crowded, but I was able to get a seat just a row or two from the rear. By the time the auction began, the room had an overflow with an entire row of standees along the back wall.

The afternoon session began promptly at 2:00 P.M. with the female auctioneer starting off at a rapid pace. One side of the room was a row of telephone operators ready to take bids from absentee bidders. Picture after picture was auctioned at rather high prices I thought. At the end, each winner was invited to hold up his or her paddle, so that the auctioneer could announce the lot number followed by the price, and winner's paddle number.

At last the auctioneer said the next lot would be Number 187, titled "The Factory" by Alfred Stieglitz. This was apparently the item many had been waiting for. It was an eleven by fourteen inch black and white photograph of a factory scene with smoke stacks emitting clouds of gray smoke from their chimneys, mounted in a simple black wooden frame with a white three inch matting.

It amazed me that anything could be listed at such a high price. But then again how could a Van Gogh painting of sunflowers be auctioned at over $20 million dollars or, an oil painting of his psychiatrist for $40 million? (On second thought anything having to do with psychiatry is overpriced these days.)

In any case, it would be interesting to see what this photograph will actually sell for. The very professional looking and well-dressed lady auctioneer in her forties stepped up to the microphone and said,

"We will begin the bidding for "The Factory" at $50,000."

I gasped. How could this be? I thought. After all, this is only a photograph, but the bidding climbed at a rapid clip of $10,000 dollars each time an arm moved or a paddle was flashed.

In a few minutes the bids had flown past $100,000. Since I was sitting in the rear I could see many of the interested bidders from all over the room, as well as the panel of telephone bids.

It was apparent that there was a great deal of interest in "The Factory", but as the bids drew closer to the $200,000 level there were fewer and fewer active participants. As the price went higher the auctioneer invited larger increments. Now the bids were increasing at the rate of $25,000 dollars!

When the bidding had passed $300,000 dollars, I realized that there were only two bidders actively giving bids at this level.

The auctioneer would not give the number, but just say,

"We have a bid of $325,000 sitting on the right side in the rear of the room."

Then she said, "$350,000 is standing in the back of the room." As she said that, I suddenly saw the person who had bid. She was a tall woman in a black suit, and had just touched her right hand to her left elbow, this must have been her well-known sign.

Then, as I turned around toward the front, the auctioneer said, "Do we have a bid of $375,000?" I saw a woman in a gray business suit just in front of me put her right hand up to her right ear.

I was amazed to think I now knew the two bidders who were involved in this titanic struggle of modern day gladiators. I understand professional bidders do not want anyone to know that they are bidding. Hence, the auctioneers do not give away the identity of the bidder in such an important contests.

All of a sudden I heard the auctioneer say, "We have a $400,000 bid in the rear.

I turned around to see her right hand on her left elbow. Sure enough, I was right. It was the lady in black standing in the rear who bid the $400,000.

Now the auctioneer says, "Will anyone make it $425,000?"

The room was quiet. Nobody moved, except those who turned around to get a glimpse of possible bidders. I noticed that everyone was being careful not to give the auctioneer the idea that a movement of a head or hand could be an actual bid. Even I was careful not to make any overt moves that may cause a lot of embarrassment.

But we need not to worry because the auctioneer knew all the possible participants very well. She knew where to look and who the important people in this contest were.

The lady in gray in front of me was no doubt one of the big players. I suddenly saw her put her right hand to her right ear, and almost simultaneously the auctioneer said, "We have a bid of $425,000 sitting in the rear on the right." Yes! I was right. That lady certainly was the bidder. This was such great fun. I was hoping she would win.

"Who will make it $450,000?" sounds out the lady auctioneer as she looked around the room. It is now clear that the bidding was down to two bidders. The lady in front of me whose signal was to put her right hand to her right ear, and the tall woman in the black dress who stood in the back of the room, who puts her right hand across to her left elbow when she signals. This was great excitement, especially since I knew for certain the identity of the players.

"Yes, we have a $450,000 bid standing in the back of the room. Who will make it $475,000?"

The entire gallery was silent. The auctioneer continued to gaze around the room including the telephone board to make sure she was not missing a quiet bidder.

The auctioneer repeated, "We have $450." (Now she began to leave off the "thousands" because it was obvious.)

"Who will make it $475?"

"Are we done? Is there another bid?" she questioned.

The auctioneer now looks directly at the lady in front of me.

I thought, "Is she by any chance looking at me?" I did not move a muscle in the rare possibility that she would say, "We have a new bidder, a man in the next to the last row on the right" while I passed out.

But my instant daydream/nightmare disintegrated, as she said, "Going once. Fair warning…"

All of a sudden, "We have a lady's bid of $475,000 sitting on the right side!" The auctioneer hesitated to give everyone a chance to absorb this huge amount of money being offered for a black and white picture. I am further relieved that she said "lady's bid and not gentleman's bid." My quickee daydream did not materialize into reality.

"Is there a $500,000 bid?" The auctioneer was a patient woman. There was much tension around the room as everyone looked for potential bidders. The half million dollar landmark bid might have encouraged other bidders. Also, no black and white photo had ever gone for this much money. Everyone sat patiently waiting with the auctioneer.

Then all of a sudden she says, "We have $500,000 for "The Factory" as if she had to remind everyone why they were here. The bidder is standing in the rear of the room.

Then she says, "Who will make it $525?"

Again, the gallery is deathly quiet.

The auctioneer repeats, "We have $500, is there a $525 bid?"

The gallery is quiet again.

"Is there a final bid?" she asks.

"Going once (pause). Going twice (longer pause). Fair warning."

As she was about to say "Gone" she said in a high-pitched voice, "Ladies and Gentlemen, we have $525,000 sitting on the right side" just as I saw the lady in front of me slowly bring her right hand to her right ear lobe. I could see that she was really hesitant.

It was obvious that we were getting close to the end. After all, this was just a photograph, and we are now talking more than one half million dollars. I could not imagine that the bidding would get any higher. Maybe my friend in the gray suit in front of me would actually get it.

My heart was pounding, when I heard the auctioneer say, "$550,000 is the bid from the very persistent lady in the black dress standing in the rear." It was a quick bid and I could tell from its speed and the auctioneer's tone that it came from a bidder who was not going to be denied.

Once again the room was quiet. Then the auctioneer said, "We have the bid at $550,000!" she says emphatically. "Is there a bid for $575,000?" Quiet. Minutes seem to drag by.

"Do we have any further bidding at this time?" Quiet.

"Going once." The room is still. I look at my lady friend in front of me. She is staring off in the distance.

"Going twice." Said the auctioneer as she looks around the room, and glances in our direction. Neither the lady in front of me nor I show any apparent interest. We are actually intensely interested, but do not show it. After all, we are sophisticated bidders. Alright, she in reality, and me in fantasy.

It was near the end of a very difficult competition. Because she was sitting so close to me, I had allied myself with her, and darn it, we were losing. I suddenly found myself saying under my breath, "Go for another $25,000" but she did not hear my plea.

"Fair warning" the auctioneer (who also fortunately does not hear me) says again for the final time.

"Gone!" as the gavel comes down with sharp CRACK.

The entire room breaks out in a round of spontaneous applause and after a moment or two, the tension is eased. The battle of the bidding titans was over. At that moment the auctioneer returns to her very formal composure and states,

"Lot 187, "The Factory by Alfred Stieglitz is sold to paddle XXX for $550,000. Thank you ladies and gentlemen. We will move on to Lot 188."

I picked up my cane and walked to the door having witnessed the highest amount of money ever paid for a photograph. I suddenly realized that my hands were sweating. I have seen exciting horse races and tennis matches, but the excitement of this competition beat them all. I have viewed a lot of Alfred Stieglitz pictures at the Met, but no presentation ever had the dramatics of this one.

As I walked down the block I wondered where "The Factory" was actually going to reside tonight.

3. GETTING SCAMMED

Recently there was an article on the Internet about the ten worst scams in the country. Some had to do with construction jobs, or auto repairs, then there were some involving credit cards and telephone services. At the end of the article it stated how people often got scammed and did not tell about it because they were embarrassed to tell others about being taken. After reading that, I realized that I fell into that category. It is just down right embarrassing to have been scammed, and you do not want people to know how dumb, greedy or foolish you were when you were taken for a ride. I have been writing stories for almost ten years now and I never thought about writing how I got scammed.

I think the only way that many scams will get stopped is if the people who get scammed admit it and talk openly about it, so that others will not make the same mistake.

The feeling is terrible. You feel angry and abused. You want the person who did it to get punished and suffer some outrageous penalty. Of course you never think about blaming yourself, but I guess that is just human nature. One of the instincts I had was to not to talk about it at all.

So in a way, this is an open confession about how I got taken, and after five years I am ready to go public and admit to my foolishness and to my greed in getting scammed. One of the main reasons I want to talk publicly is so that others will not make the same mistake.

One of the first things that I asked when I found out that I was scammed is that it happened to so many others. Some how it felt a little better when I found out that there were about ten thousand others. I guess misery does like company.

For about twenty-five years I have been investing with mostly one broker who is paid full commission to buy both stocks and bonds.

I did not do too well. I never made any great killings, but did not do too badly either. In retrospect, I suppose I would be called an average investor. My investments were in the age before the Internet boom when thousands of people lost their fortunes in what many investors now consider legal scams during the past three years.

But getting back to my real scam, it was the kind that gets written about The New York Times. One day I received a call from a broker who sounded really nice and legitimate. He had several investments for my consideration. They were small companies, the kind that my old time broker would not even recommend. This broker who called me charged about one-half of the commission I had been paying.

I was very cautious and spoke to him three or four times, prior to making a small investment. To this day I do not know the reason I finally opened up a small account with him, nevertheless I did. In the past I had gotten dozens of calls from similar brokers, but never considered them. This time somehow or other, I bought stock. Now this man seemed very honest, and I realized that is the way one often gets caught. The stock that he recommended was a small growth stock, and in the six months that I had it, it did go up. In retrospect, if he had recommended a dud, it would have been the best thing that could have happened to me, but it went up in addition to a few others he recommended. I consider myself a very cautious investor, and put about sixty percent of my money in stocks, and the rest in bonds.

Over a period of two or three years I gradually developed a portfolio with Mr. New Broker, but never cut out Mr. Old Broker. Even with Mr. New Broker I felt that I should split my portfolio between stocks and bonds. I thought that this was just the safe way to invest.

Now Mr. New Broker was a member of a small-size brokerage house, not big enough to clear their stocks and bonds themselves, they did it through another company. This did not seem too suspicious because hundreds of little companies do just that. Over the first three years I developed a portfolio of stocks and bonds with Mr. New Broker that was about 25% of my assets.

Then one day I mentioned to Mr. New Broker that the interest rate on the bonds that he was selling me was going down from about 7% to about 5.5%. Mr. New Broker said he had a new group of bonds that were backed by local school districts, and paid 7% to 7.5%; this was much better than the regular bonds that city and states paid. Wow! I thought this was great. These bonds in effect were paying almost 40% more than I was getting from either Mr. Old broker or Mr. New Broker.

I received a lot of information about the school districts and townships that were selling these bonds. They seemed legitimate enough, and even paid interest on a monthly basis. Even so, I was cautious about it and only bought one bond.

I said to Mr. New Broker. "Let's see how this works out." Now Mr. New Broker was never a high-pressure salesman. He never pushed me very hard to buy more and more. As I look back over the years, it was a perfect set-up. No high pressure, lots of legitimate sales. Everything looked great. Every month I would get checks for the principal and interest. So each time that I received several months of money back, I liked the deal so much that I encouraged Mr. New Broker to look into more bonds like this. Over two or three years I gradually built quite a portfolio of these great bonds that paid two or so points over the going rate of the market.

Then, one day Mr. New Broker called to tell me that the company issuing these bonds would not be sending out the principal and interest payments this month. He said they were a little short on cash. They would only send out the interest payments for the next few months. "But do not worry, this would be straightened out in the next few months. And by the way did I want to buy any other bonds at this time?"

At least I was smart enough not to buy any more of those bonds. A month later The New York Times had an article about my investment company, and that the FBI and SEC had subpoenaed their records. The next morning Mr. New Broker called to tell me he had some very bad news. He told me that thousands of these bonds were found to be worthless and that the investment company had sold the same computers to the same school districts four and five times. In essence, there was no value behind the bonds. Over the couple of years I was involved with this company they had set up a scam where thousands of investors had bought worthless paper. The Bennett family (actual name) had scammed over ten thousand investors with a fraudulent scheme that sold the same item many times. As the scheme unfolded, it was disclosed that many people invested all their savings in this company.

I began to hear how medical companies and nursing associations put all their investments in those deals. Other people invested all their pension assets in the scheme. The stories I heard got worse and worse. As I read more about this scheme, I learned that more and more people were taken for all they were worth. I was relieved that I had not been taken for more money.

Of course, the court appointed a trustee, Mr. Richard Breeden, former head of the SEC, to oversee the case. Lawyers came out of the woodwork from every corner of the state requesting to represent me and the other defrauded investors. The trustee, Mr. Breedon, was an excellent and honest lawyer who worked hard for three years to help get our money back. The big question was what happened to almost one billion dollars of hard earned invested funds?

One investigation after another turned up illegal hotels, racetracks, yachts, and Swiss bank accounts. Five years later and hundreds of hours of lawyer manpower, and we have gotten some of our investment back. At least eight people were sent to prison from two to thirty years. Unfortunately Mrs. Bennett had many of the assets in her name, so they could not pin the fraud on her.

When the judge handed down Patrick Bennett's sentence, the judge stated that a horrible crime was committed against the little investor in the State of New

York. He handed down an interesting verdict. Mr. Bennett had the option of a twenty-year prison sentence if his wife voluntarily returned all of her ill-received gains, like the hotel and racetrack or a thirty-year sentence if she does not give them back. Mrs. Bennett was given thirty days to make her decision.

When the thirty days were over Mrs. Bennett came to court and said that she would keep all the property. So, Mr. Bennett was given the thirty-year sentence (what a loving wife, I thought.) In any case, the Trustee, Mr. Breedon, is still going after these assets. The Bennett parents were forced to return the yacht, while other family members had to sell various assets like the country clubs, motels, and racehorses.

During the last five years I have slowly received only about 28% of my investment back, and have agonized thinking about this experience every time I get one of those little checks.

The one big lesson I learned from all of this, is when something is too good to be true, it is usually not.

4. FAVORITE GARDENS AROUND THE WORLD

Victoria, British Columbia
Christchurch, New Zealand
Charleston, South Carolina
Martinique, Caribbean
Kyoto, Japan
Botanical Park, Montreal
Central Park, New York

Seven gardens plus one for good measure (My Little Garden World)

Today I am going to share stories with you about my favorite gardens. They are spread around our planet, and, as you will see, have very different personalities. From Canada to New Zealand, from Japan, to the Caribbean come fly with me on a magic carpet of lovely blooms.

Victoria, British Columbia

The first garden that comes to mind is found in the neighbor country to the north. It is in the city of Victoria in the territory of British Columbia. It is approximately 20 miles from this quaint city that is similar to many cities in old England. The garden is called Buschard Gardens, and had its beginnings in a very ignominious way. For several years the owner of the property used the soil and dirt of construction projects around British Columbia. After using all the dirt that he needed, the end result was a huge hole several hundreds of acres across. His wife had the idea of turning this eye sore into something a lot more beautiful; therefore a picturesque international garden arose from this hole in the ground.

She went all around the world buying plants, trees, and flowers to develop the garden of her dreams. She divided the area into gardens of different nations, about six in all. Each one is prettier than the next. The English garden is quaint and typical of an English country side. The oriental garden has Japanese miniature red maples and many different types of Bonsai plants. An Italian country garden has also a complete Roman vineyard. There are streams and brooks with water lilies in bloom.

I wish I knew how to put video pictures on the e mail so that I could show them to you. You would be thrilled to see these incredible beautiful flowers in full bloom. We spent a whole day in the Buschard gardens and the time flow by as we enjoyed it tremendously. The tulips, narcissus, azalea and hundreds of other species were a thrill to enjoy.

We walked over the wooden bridges and across the lawns having a great time at this never-to be-forgotten garden of my dreams.

Christchurch, New Zealand

Traveling diagonally across the Pacific, we landed in the small but elegant little city of about one hundred thousand people on the South Island of New Zealand called Christchurch. We arrived there on the 25th of October in the middle of spring.

I am sure you remember that in the southern hemisphere the seasons are reversed. All the lawns, shrubs and trees were in their fullest color. A river slowly meanders through this city of dreams. On the river are white boats called "punts" that carry visitors around the gardens for a romantic trip on the River Avon. A punt is a type of rowboat that has a paddler standing in the rear, like a gondolier would stand in the rear of the gondolier in the Italian City of Venice. He is dressed in an immaculate white uniform including a white sporty hat and holds a long pole that propels the punt slowly down the river. The punt seats about four passengers while they enjoy their leisurely trip down the Avon. When we visited, we saw a group of teenage girls celebrating ones sixteenth birthday. It was such a happy occasion, I cannot forget this young person's innocent enjoyment of a byegone era. The park also has two passenger kayak boats enjoyed by the children of the city. I appreciated this fun and relaxed type of park.

Christchurch has a very different pace from Queenstown, where tourists can take exciting trips on jet boats, leap off high bridges by means of bungie cords, and land in the center of the city by way of paragliding. But getting back to Christchurch and its beauty, Lila and I spent two wonderful days taking videos and stills, enjoying the relaxed atmosphere in this park, and just absorbing the beauty of one of the prettiest gardens on earth. I walked among the azaleas, and gigantic rhododendrons coming into blossom, tulips were also in bloom.

One of the most impressive things I found about the park was the peace and tranquility of the entire place. Christchurch's park has earned a place as one of my favorites.

Charleston, South Carolina

With the magic of the jet age and the speed of light, I will take you half way around the earth to the East coast of the United States to the city of Charleston, South Carolina. Once again it is springtime in the Northern hemisphere.

It is the month of April with the azaleas and rhododendrons in their most gorgeous color. Charleston is a historic city that was involved in the Civil War with the famous Fort Sumter as the location of the first battle of the tragic conflict. Long before the Civil War was fought, there was a garden about ten miles from the city called Magnolia Plantation Gardens.

Lila and I drove out to the gardens and were immediately transfixed with the immensity of the trees, and the vibrancy of the color. There were hundreds of huge stately looking trees that form the background of this extraordinary park. We walked through the lanes and down the paths, over the wooden bridges and upon observation decks. The color in every direction was just spectacular. We spent hours looking at the shrubs and at the monuments to the family members who lived in this area for three centuries. It has been ten years since I drove into that pretty city, but I still remember its gardens as one of the prettiest.

It is very interesting to me that every garden can have its own personality, just as people have their personality. For example, an English type of garden is very neat and well-kept similar to the one in Christchurch. The garden in Charleston was more rustic with wooden bridges and curved paths lined with azaleas. Then, one can also enjoy tropical gardens such as the one on the island of Martinique known as the Jarden de Balata.

Martinique in the Caribbean

Our ship anchored in the harbor of Martinique at Port de France. We walked through the local market and bought a coconut on the way out to the gardens. Instead of taking a tour of the island, we decided to just hop on a local bus to visit the gardens on our own. It was only a ten-minute ride to a wonderful, tropical paradise that is so very different from a neat English garden.

It was a little like a jungle, except with paths and signs. There were huge trees and shrubs that in some cases had leaves twelve inches across. They had philodendron plants similar to one we have in our kitchen, but theirs were triple the size, possibly fifteen feet high. They also had magnificent bird-of-paradise plants that seemed to grow wild all around us. One was similar to the type we have in our greenhouse in Hauppauge, New York. I celebrate if my bird-of-paradise gets one flower in a season, but in Martinique there were flowering bird-of-paradise plants all over.

All of a sudden we saw a pair of bright green hummingbirds flapping their wings at an incredible speed as they sipped nectar from one of the many tropical plants. It was an exciting sight. Both Lila and I took pictures and shot videos in this dreamlike setting; hours went by like minutes. Suddenly Lila looked at her watch, and said "It is late. We had better get going." We reluctantly left the Jarden de Balata. On the way back to the ship, I bought a large poster which still hangs up in my den depicting this garden.

Fortunately we jumped on a bus just in time to get the last tender going back to our sailing ship for the week, The Windstar. We set sail almost immediately to the island of St. Lucia for the next day's wonderful experience.

Kyoto, Japan

Let's fly across the Pacific Ocean once again as I would like to introduce you to a very different type of garden. So far we have seen formal English gardens, tropical gardens, and variety gardens, but the most unusual of all gardens are those in the city of Kyoto, Japan. It is in that city where you will view magnificent stone and pebble gardens. These Zen gardens are ornate in a very different way, because they do not have growing plants or flowers, but instead are simple rocks of different shapes and sizes, surrounded by combed pebbles.

The garden that I liked best was one called Ryoan-ji. The garden is approximately 40 meters by 10 meters (110 feet by 30 feet) in a rectangle shape. As you walk around the periphery, you are instructed to count the rocks that sit majestically in their pebble setting, somewhat like shrubs on a lawn. This may appear to be a simple task indeed, but no matter how many times one counts the rocks, they always add up to fourteen. However, you are given the fact that there are fifteen stones in the garden. There always seems to be one stone you can never see. That is the intriguing part of this garden.

No matter how sure one can be of something, there may be times when we just do not know what we think we know. That is the message of this very intriguing garden. It is an interesting philosophy, and really gets people to think. Besides the thinking aspect of these gardens, they also have a very simple beauty. I walked away quietly absorbing the message I had just been given, as well as enjoying the beauty and elegant simplicity I was fortunate enough to observe.

Montreal's Botanical Gardens

At the end of a twelve-day cruise along the northeastern portion of the USA and Canada, my cousin Joe and I spent the last three days in Montreal. It was a wonderful trip going from New York, to Newport, Rhode Island, and then up along the Maritime Provinces and then to Quebec and Montreal.

I had a map brochure of Montreal, and one of the places that often popped up was its Botanical Gardens, so we decided to visit them. When we arrived we saw signs all over the gardens announcing the Chinese lantern exhibition for the next two weeks. Luckily, we were there just at the right time. The Botanical Gardens are so huge, that the only way to see all of it is to take their mini-bus.

We got off at the Chinese exhibition and started to walk around. In the center of the man-made lake were hundreds of paper mache figures of sailing boats, fishermen, fish and dozens of other figures of fruit and animals, just too spectacular to believe. Among the paper mache figures were hundreds of Chinese lanterns with dozens of Bonsai plants from two hundred to five hundred years old that added to the overall beauty. Even though we took the mini-bus, the Chinese section was so large that I became tired from walking within this one section.

But when I am interested in something I just overcome my pain, and keep on going. We got back on the tram and went to the Japanese section. There were magnificent indoor and outdoor gardens that I would not have missed for the world. We spent another hour or two there, but I was exhausted by the end of the day.

When it comes to gardens, I just cannot give up, so we traveled to the other end of the park to the United States western exhibitions. The garden had dozens of Bonsai, some as ancient as eight hundred years old. They also had western ponderosa pines in Bonsai form that were impressive. I could not make up my mind to choose between the Chinese, Japanese or western American Bonsai exhibitions as my favorite.

The one thing that I knew for sure was that I had to add the Montreal Botanical Gardens to my list of favorites.

Central Park, N.Y.

You have now read about six gardens from around the world and I hope you have enjoyed them. We will fly back on our magic carpet, and before you know it we are home walking in our own Central Park that has a garden in it as beautiful as any around the world. In the middle of one of the largest concentration of humans on earth, Central Park has a special little corner called, "A Secret Garden" just a mile or so from my apartment. It is a garden unknown to most people because it is fenced in with only one entrance on Fifth Avenue that one cannot enter from the park itself. But it is carefully groomed so that some flowers are continually in bloom from March to October. One afternoon I was walking through my little secret garden when I saw a lady bending down to pick up a leaf.

I started a conversation with her in my typical friendly way, I said, "Isn't this a beautiful place? and it is so well kept that I am surprised you even found a leaf to pick up." She stood up and said to me, "Oh! Thank you, I am glad you like it." I did not understand her thanks, until she told me that she was the chief horticulturist of "A Secret Garden."

I discovered a person so interested in her job and so loving of the flowers she planted that she felt I deserved a "Thank You" for noticing her work. The woman then shared how much care her little garden took, how she chose the various flowers, and which species she picked so that one would bloom continually throughout the year. As she talked I could see that her heart and soul was in this little place with the love she showed to every bud and leaf.

I was amazed to hear her talk about this garden in the middle of one of the largest city on earth, as if it were her own personal garden. The Secret Garden was her and she was the Secret Garden. I found that the secret was her love for the garden. I thought of all the gardens around the world that I have seen, and realized that each of them must have someone just like that little lady in Central Park kneeling down to pick up a single leaf. The secret to every garden is the people who bend down to pick up each leaf and smell each flower.

One for good measure: My Little Garden World

Although I have had wonderful times viewing gardens around the world, there was one little garden that has for thirty-three years held a special place in my heart. When I have suffered in pain or frustration I could always sit on my lounge and look at my own special garden. When my wife and I chose the location of our house, I was especially careful to pick the property that had the most beautiful trees; I love shady gardens with lots of tall trees.

Each year my wife and kids purchased a special tree or shrub for me on Father's Day to add to the natural greenery of the property. We have added to the beauty of our home by enhancing it with lovely trees from miniature Japanese red maples to magnificent copper beeches. We also planted crab apples, flowering plums, pink dogwood, azaleas, Rhododendron of many colors and varieties. One year my family bought me a rare shrub called a Harry Lauder's walking stick. It is a very unusual shrub with knurled branches that grow to a height of about eight feet. It was named after a famous comedian who lived in the early twentieth century who walked around with a crocked cane that resembled the shrub. (Sadly this tree died last year) In addition to these lovely specimens given to me on Father's Day, I have treated myself with special miniature evergreens that have become a unique part of my property.

This little garden is less than thirty feet long and ten feet wide, but it holds a very special place in my heart; it is my favorite little garden. It is less than one percent of the property, but is loaded with pretty little plants and rocks that I have collected from all over the world. I call it my "Little Garden World" because when I visit places I bring home miniature plants or specimen rocks, and add them lovingly to this little garden. In one corner, there are rocks from Utah or Arizona's Grand Canyon. I brought home colorful little rocks from as far away as Canada's Yukon Territory or Australia's Ayers Rock.

Over the years, I have added a Chinese Pagoda, a Japanese Statue, and a replica of an old wooden bridge to the garden. In the last two years I have received intriguing granite signs each with a single contemplative word, namely, "wonder" and "inspiration."

I love to sit by my garden and imagine I am traveling throughout the world, seeing all those wondrous places. At times when the pain has limited my ability to travel as far as I would like to, I can sit by my garden, and let my imagination take me to those far-off places.

5. REMEMBERING THE TOWERS

It has been over two years since all New Yorkers experienced the worst tragedy in our history. Until today, I have not written a story remembering my many visits to the Towers. September 11th was a terrible morning as I rushed between the window of our living room and the TV room where I was getting an all too vivid view of what was happening downtown. From my living room I could see the smoke rising across the entire southern exposure of our apartment. The sky was dark with smoke and air filled with dust. I hardly ever look out my living room view without thinking of that terrible morning.

Now it is two years later, and I am once again letting myself think of better days when I experienced many visits to the World Trade Center. When I wanted to impress customers or friends with the elegance of our city, I would always take them to the Windows On the World at the top of one of the Twin Towers. Without question, Windows on the World has the finest view of any restaurant in the world. I have many fond memories of the times we spent there, and no terrorist bomb can take them from me.

My first exciting experience was the view I got looking north or uptown to the Empire State Building. I arrived a few minutes before my visitors and decided to take a self-guided tour. The sky was clear and bright and looking down upon the city below was absolutely thrilling. To think that one could actually be looking down on the Empire State Building was almost unbelievable. For almost my entire life, the Empire State Building was the tallest building on earth. Now I was looking down upon it and all the other buildings in the city; it was and still is a sight I shall never forget.

Then I walked around to the other side of the cocktail lounge to see lower New York harbor, home of the Statue of Liberty, Staten Island Ferry, Verrazano Bridge, and the bright lights of Manhattan's Wall Street skyscrapers. From the entrance of the restaurant I also saw the five East River bridges from the Brooklyn Bridge and its spectacular nineteenth century architecture to the Triborough Bridge and its modern day suspension style in the North.

I remember that first night our representative from Greece, Costa Costantanetes was coming from Athens. Now Costa was a world traveler for sure, so I wanted to impress him with New York's best. Naturally we went to the Windows on the World. We had a wonderful time that evening. We talked about many places in the United States we had visited. I told him that one of my favorite cities was New Orleans and I tried to remember a famous jazz group I had seen in that old city. I was shocked when Costa said, "Oh you must mean "Preservation

Hall." He even remembered the name of the pianist called Grandma Emma. It amazed me that he had such a worldwide range of musical knowledge.

We sat looking out at the city as I thought of the comparable view in Costa's city, Athens and it's Acropolis. It is hard to believe that Costa told me about the night the Turks had all but destroyed that magnificent monument about seven centuries ago. However, the Greeks rebuilt it, and the Parthenon still stands in the heart of Athens on top of its hill, the Acropolis. Little did I know that a similar, but much more destructive fate would befall our towers.

Another visit to the Windows was to celebrate our son Marc's engagement to Meg. Lila and I thought it would be nice to invite Meg's parents and our children to the Windows. I called a few days ahead for a window table reservation. We arrived at the Towers and took the elevator to the 110th floor. I was surprised that for once the elevators were not crowded. We got off and went to the restaurant side. Again, I was surprised that although it was a Saturday night, the place was not crowded. When we walked into the restaurant, I was shocked that it appeared as though the shades had been pulled down. Suddenly I realized that the clouds had pulled a complete curtain around the windows. I had not been sophisticated enough to check the cloud ceiling before going to the Windows On The World. Later I found out that the ceiling was about five hundred feet that evening. Apparently, many people cancel their reservations when the view is not going to be worthwhile. What a disappointment. From then on I always checked the cloud ceiling before going to the Windows.

On several other occasions I went to the Windows with Naval officers to honor special milestones on our major program for the P-3 aircraft. The last dinner at the Windows was a rather unpleasant one for me. There were about ten of us enjoying a very pleasant dinner when all of a sudden I became dizzy, and felt as though I needed to lay down.

I was taken to a couch and one of my associates called for an Emergency Medical Team. I felt very uncomfortable, as well as quite embarrassed for causing such a stir. When the EMT arrived they wanted to take me to the hospital, but by that time I was feeling better so I decided to just go home and rest. I believed that it was a combination of too much alcohol combined with the high altitude that affected my blood sugar level. This incident was also pivotal in determining my hypoglycemia.

That was my last trip to the World Trade Center, and my final remembrance of the Windows On The World, until that is, September 11th 2001.

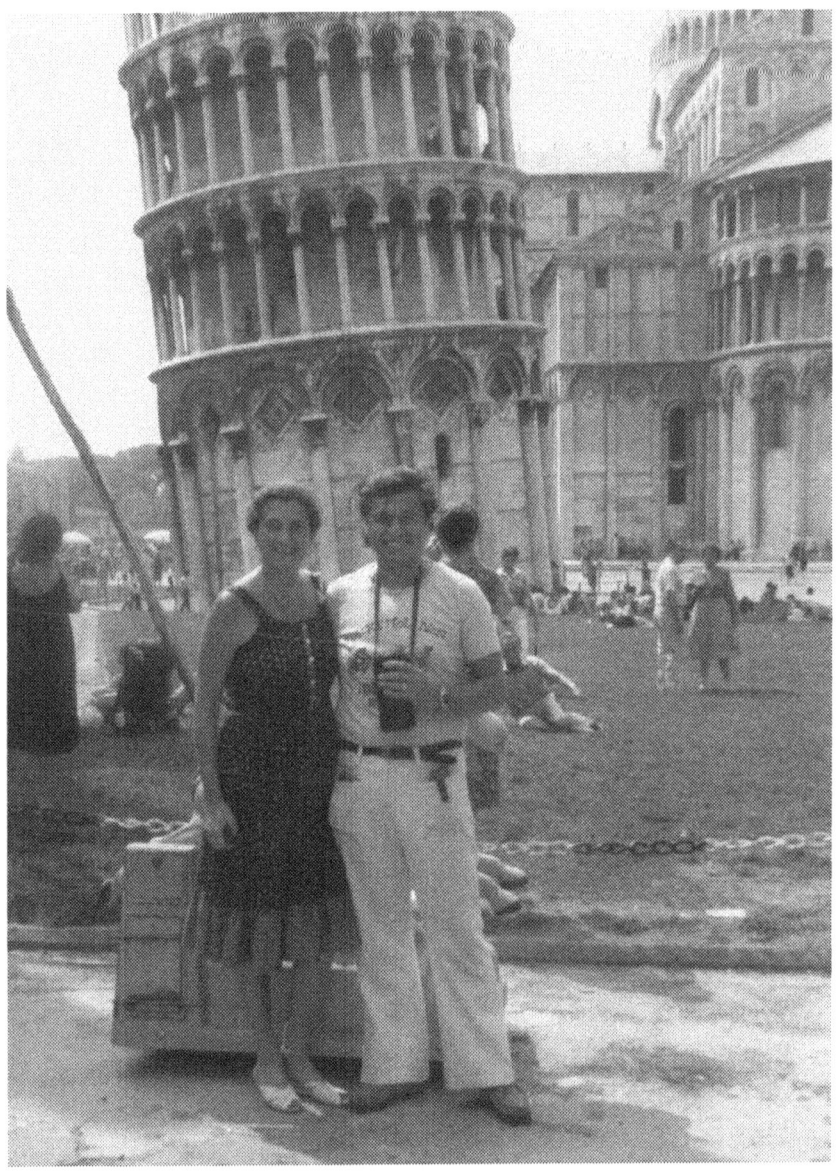

Lila and Gene Traveling in Pisa

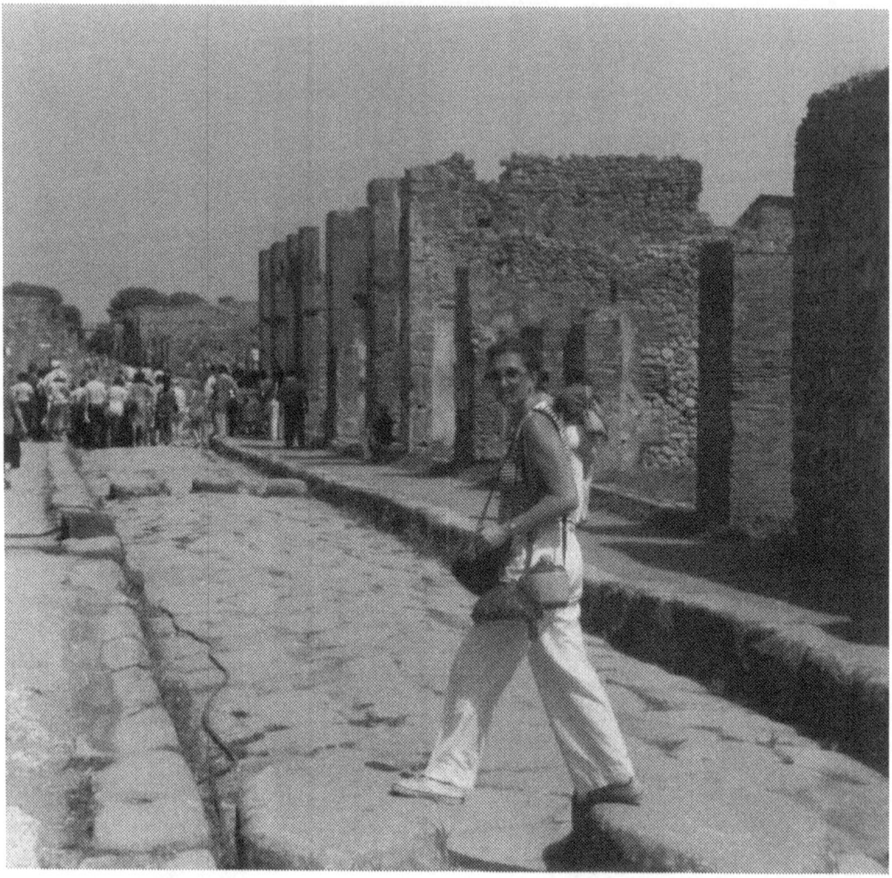

Lila Crossing the Steppingstones of Pompeii

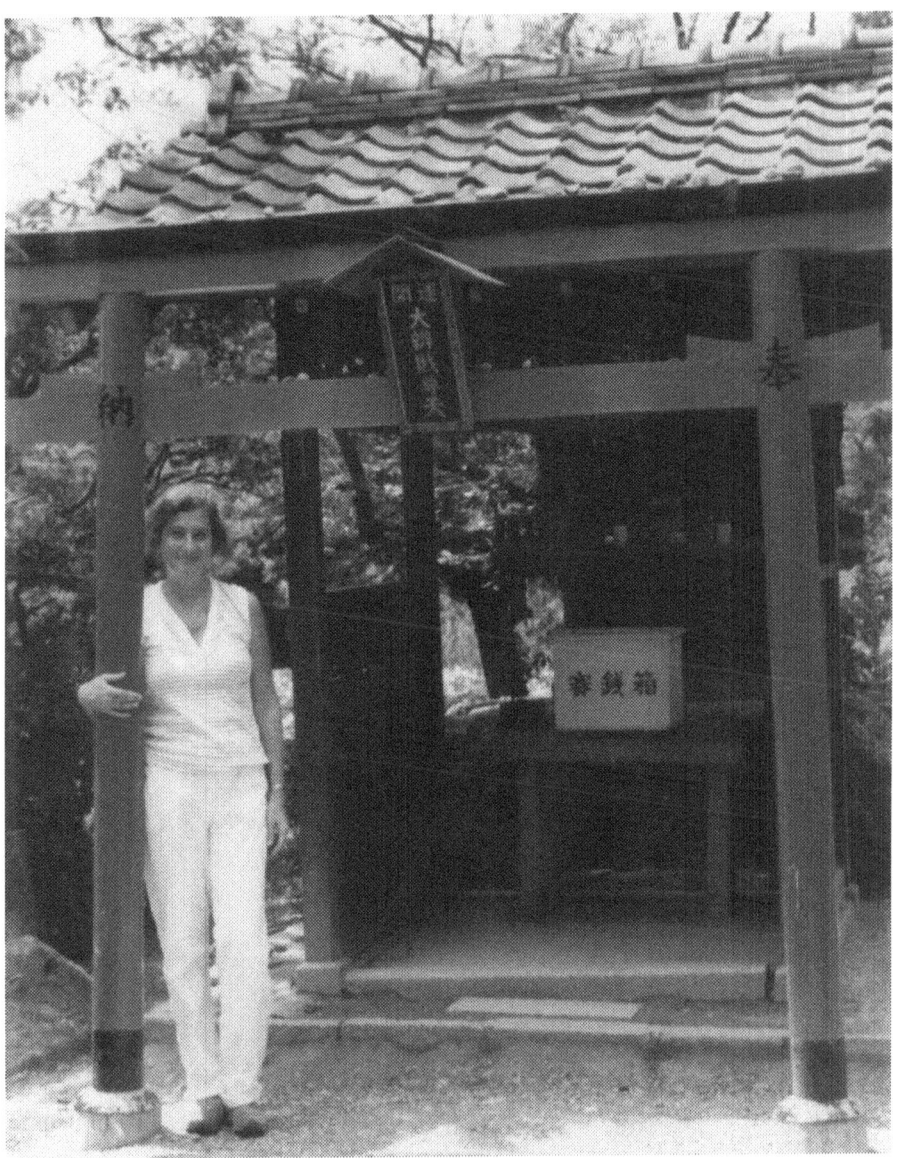

Lila in Kyoto, Japan

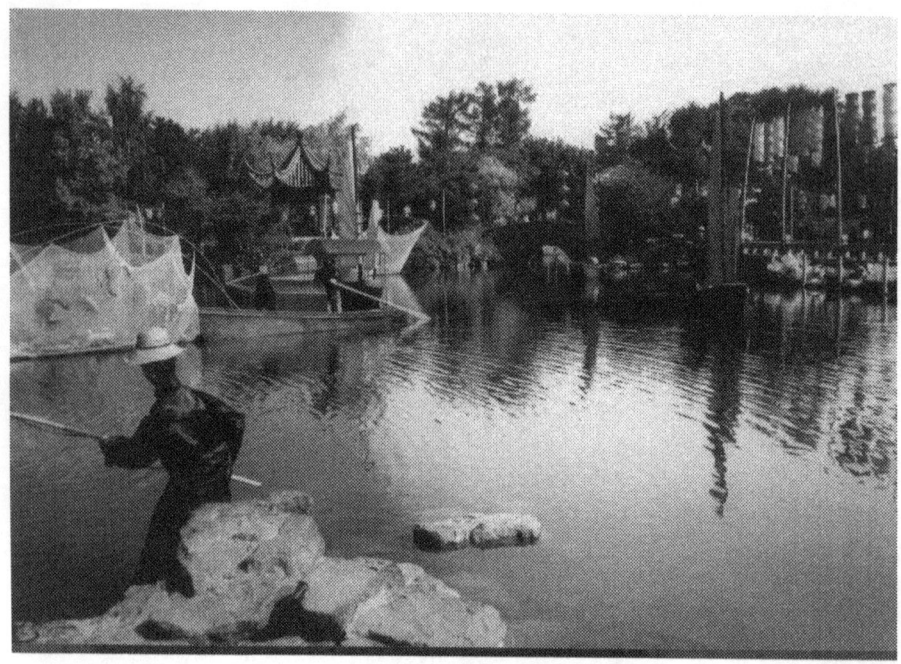

Chinese Garden, Montreal

Final Chapter

Dedicated to my wife Lila

1. Surprisingly Fun Times

All Work and No Play Makes Gene a Dull Boy

During the twenty years as a General Manager, I put a lot of effort to make my division a place where our workers could be proud to call it their second home. After all, it was my belief that one spent more waking hours at work, than in his or her own home. I loved my place of work and wanted my fellow workers to feel the same way. Shortly after I took over, I encouraged people to make General Instrument a career place to spend their years.

I set up programs to give awards for years of service. We set up a special program for everyone who worked in our company for twenty-five years to be given medals. Each year we would have a dinner to honor those workers with twenty-five years of service. At that dinner, everyone who had worked at GI for a significant length of time would be honored equally. The dinner gave everybody equal recognition from Leroy the Porter to Al, a model maker who was there for forty years.

The first year we had the party only ten people were eligible, but over the ensuing years we had fifty-five workers who were employed for twenty-five years or more. We also gave gold pins to employees who were there in multiplies of five years. The division's walls had plaques with the names of all who were at GI in five, ten, fifteen, or twenty years. To encourage excellent workmanship we would choose an employee of the month who would be honored with a picture and an article in the division newspaper.

It was clear that milestones were important and enjoyable times for both Lila and myself. At every milestone in my life she was there with a fun and memorable experience. As I look back over my life there are three that are very significant.

2. My 50th Birthday

All three of these experiences were Lila's ideas and were completely orchestrated by her. In December of 1976, I had been a General Manager for four exciting years. When I took over the reins in 1972, Irving Kaufman had resigned without much warning, to work as General Manager of Page Communication. It was unusual for an executive to leave with short notice, but Irv's new company wanted him there in less than a month. How I got the job is described in the tale called "The Inside Story of Becoming the G.M." It took several long years to turn the ship around, but by 1975 we were making money with the hard work and dedication of a great staff.

When my fiftieth birthday rolled around, Lila decided that I should have a party with all my staff as well as other friends, and that it should be a surprise. I was too busy with work to think about my upcoming birthday. On a Saturday night a week before my birthday, we went out for a usual dinner with friends. We came back around 8:00 P.M. and I did not the slightest idea that fifty people were lurking in our living room.

Lila had skillfully arranged for guests to park their cars at the end of our street. When we came back from dinner, I remember making a casual comment, "It looks like somebody was having a party up the block." Never thinking that those cars belonged to my friends.

I walked into a darkened house to be completely surprised by a mob of family and friends. I was so surprised that tears came to my eyes. What a shock! I was taken back with one highlight after another. The kids all wrote and recited a poem that described their feelings for me. Each of my staff gave me a present, but one gift stands out as so very special. The director of Quality Assurance, Al, handed me a big box and I could not imagine what in the world it could be. I opened it and read the accompanying card. The gift was a huge train tunnel from a model railroad set. He wrote, "Now we can see the light at the end of the tunnel." After almost four years of hard work this was such an appropriate gift now that we were making money and having a good time to boot.

Then, another big package was given to me. It was a huge card drawn by the company artist, Al Mazzola, signed by roughly six hundred employees of the Long Island and Boston divisions.

Al had a way of drawing the greatest cards, but of course the ideas were Lila's.

Each year I would have a grand birthday celebration coincide with the company's annual year-end party. I always expected to have a big cake as part of the dinner dance. These parties were so much fun, and I must admit I loved being the center of attraction.

Al's wonderful cards came along with the cake signed by those hundreds of great people. The spirit at Government Systems was just great. Five years after I retired, I remember meeting Ron Myer, a Program Manager of the Hellenic Air Force program, on a street in Athens where he mentioned how wonderful it was to have worked for me. Even twelve years after my retirement I will meet someone from the company who tell me how great it was to have together.

3. RETIREMENT PARTY

In 1991 I retired after thirty-nine exciting years at General Instrument/Radio Receptor, just five months before my sixty-fifth birthday. It was a logical time to retire since the Group had been sold to Litton Industries during that summer. Even though it was a hectic period, I still managed to arrange for a safari with Lila and some family members.

One fine Sunday afternoon toward the end of September as the reality of retirement was slowly sinking in, Lila said, "let's take a walk on Sunken Meadow Beach today. I always loved to walk along the Sunken Meadow boardwalk. It is one of my favorite places in our local area because the beach faces Connecticut and Long Island Sound, even though it is not as dramatic as the Atlantic Ocean.

I had not done anything all week and was feeling stir crazy because retirement had been a difficult transition for me. The idea that I would get up and not have some exciting activity or meeting for the day was hard for me to accept. Looking back on those days, I would have been so much happier if I only knew about writing, but it would be five more years and a bout with cancer to get me into this next phase of life.

We drove to the beach and Lila suggested we park at the furthest end of the park. This was not too unusual since it was less crowded there. When we started to walk on the boardwalk I noticed the beach was almost entirely empty. She then suggested "Won't it be nice to walk along the water?" to which I readily agreed. It was a beautiful sunny day with warm and comfortable weather for the end of summer.

I was thinking about how fortunate we were to be able to enjoy the day, when Lila made a strange suggestion that I walk backwards, so we could look at each other as we walked. In retrospect, I have no idea why this request did not cause any suspicion for me, but surprisingly it did not. To this day I cannot believe I was so naive. I turned around to face her and we held hands as we walked for a few hundred yards on the empty beach.

When Lila said, "How about walking straight now?"

"Okay." I replied.

I turned around to see about one hundred smiling faces yelling, "Surprise! Surprise!"

What a surprise! I felt like such a damn fool. It was a great party with marvelous food and drinks, so I traded feeling foolish for a deep appreciation of my wife's ingenuity.

4. MY 65TH BIRTHDAY

I began to do some consulting work for a little company five months after retirement because I was hanging on to my sanity by a thread. The work was very unsatisfying because I was not used to having my suggestions disregarded so off-handedly by inexperienced younger people.

I learned an interesting fact as a consultant: you did not give orders, just suggestions. In addition, one must not be too invested in getting one's ideas accepted otherwise it makes the work too frustrating. I found out that I would just supply ideas, and the bosses can choose to accept them. Eventually I concluded that consulting was not for me. Lila was at my side as I went through this frustrating time, but with her help and guidance I came out fine.

One Sunday in December while staying in our apartment in N.Y. she encouraged me to go some place for and hour or two. When I returned, there were at least thirty people all yelling, "Surprise!" I had been fooled yet again. I believe that I could so easily be fooled is that I was never expecting any of these parties and do not pay too much attention to little activities going on. For the party Lila and Danya, our niece prepared a video of pictures of my life, adding to it Lila's variation of the words of a poem called "The Station."

As I think back at those three very significant surprises in my lifetime. They all had very important messages for me to remember: Be optimistic, look for the light at the end of the tunnel, appreciate what one has and enjoy each day to the fullest and lastly, the trip is what is important and not the end.

5. A MEMORABLE TIME WITH AN EXCITING MAN

We emerged from the cab in front of the Guggenheim Museum in the spring of 2003. A nicely dressed middle-aged man with a twenty dollar bill in his hand approaches me to ask, "Do you have an extra ticket?"

"Sorry." I say. "Isn't the box office open?"

"No. It is all sold out." he says.

I was totally surprised. After all, this was not a Broadway show or a opening night for a movie. This was a poetry performance about to be given by a 98 year-old man. Why would there be two thousand people waiting on line to hear him this Sunday evening?

As we walked in, the line stretched around the entire first floor exhibition hall. We thought it would be nice to get there one half hour in advance to be sure of a front row seat. By the time we were seated, we felt lucky to be together three rows from the rear.

On the stage in a corner was a rather frail looking man with an associate. They huddled together, not overly interested in the gathering audience.

I was not too sure what to expect since I have very rarely listened to poetry readings, and have never heard of one accompanied with music. The first piece was called the Robin Redbreast. It was sung and played by a young man and a lady flutist. It was difficult to hear his falsetto tones among the shrill notes of the flute coupled with the electronic pitches of an amplifier. If this had been the level of the entire night's performance you would not be reading this story.

But, after a few poems accompanied by music, the master of ceremonies began interviewing Stanley Kunitz, past Poet Laureate of the United States.

He was just outstanding both during the interview and his reading of his poems. It was just amazing to see and hear a man approaching his centennial with such enthusiasm and vitality. His voice was clear and loud and he had incredible recall. He told us of the circumstances under which he wrote the "Robin." He remembered how, when he was fourteen, a friend gave him a gun and Stanley fired it for the very first time. It was unbelievable that he fired it into the sky and by sheer chance hit this poor bird right between the eyes. He was so affected that he sat down and wrote a poem that has become such a classic for eighty years.

The audience was mesmerized especially when he talked of the love of his garden and for gardening. He compared his garden with the stages of life, the growing up and flourishing and then finally the death. He writes with a passion and a beauty that is so compelling and touching for all those who know his works.

He told us of a story of his early days. I can sympathize with his childhood as he said his father died before he was born. It was the year 1910 and Stanley was five years old, when his Kindergarten teacher told his class that the next day an astrological phenomenon was about to take place. Haley's Comet was approaching earth and it was going to get as close as it even gets to our planet. The teacher continued saying, if the comet veers off course by a fraction of a degree it will crash into earth and we will all get destroyed. That night Stanley went to the top of his house and announced his address so that when the world was destroyed the next day, and he went to heaven, his father would know where he lived and be able to come for him. What a poignant memory for him to remember these last ninety odd years!

One special poem that is considered by many to be his best is called, "The Layers."

His favorite line is "Live in the layers and not on the litter." Kunitz' meaning of layers are the many levels of life. He encourages us to live and enjoy each one. Do not live amongst the garbage and trash of life.

As I was assembling this book, I thought of those layers he talked about this in his poem, as the chapters of my life's story. The layers for Stanley could be the sections you are reading about for me: my youth, my time in service, my career mostly at General Instrument Corp., and my illness. On further thought, possibly the illnesses was more like litter. But maybe one has to take the pain of the illness, and turn it into layers rather than litter.

"Yes!" I said to my imaginary Stanley, "my goal will be to turn the litters of the garbage pail into layers of a delicious chocolate cake."

"Yes! Lazarus, my friend, you have done it again."

I was very impressed with Stanley, first for his ideas and secondly for his ability to express them so well at the age of 98. As I left the auditorium, Lazarus said to himself, "This is my goal—to be able to think so clearly, to be able to recall my life's experiences, be able to see so well, and to be able to share my thoughts with whomever will listen to them, when I reach the ripe old age of 98."

6. SEVENTY-SEVEN YEARS

We often go to Gasho's Japan restaurant for annual celebrations like birthdays. Rachel and Matthew love to watch the cooks perform the preparation ritual with their knives. They flip them up in the air and bang them loudly on the stainless steel grill. They throw the shrimp cuttings high in the air and we cheer as they land in his ceremonial jacket or the top of the chef's hat.

After dinner the maitre d' and several waitresses come over to the table and join in the singing of the Happy Birthday song, first in English and then in Japanese. I love how they especially do the birthday song in their language. They clap twice after each line. I have no idea what they are singing, but I love how they sing it. The last line sounds like "Hapee Buthday, Grandpa."

At the end of the meal I found myself very tired. In the afternoon I had gone to the gym to exercise and I guess I had overstressed myself. Now it was not even eight o'clock and I was exhausted. It was most discouraging not to be able to spend an evening out without having to go home early. But there I was celebrating my seventy-seventh year, and feeling every bit of it. I needed assistance every bit of the way toward getting home. I needed help to put my coat on, to walk the three steps to the back door and to walk very slowly to the parking lot. There was Lila, Sharon, Matthew and Rachel all around ready to help at every turn.

On the walk out to the car Lila was on my left with her arm tightly around my waist, and I believed if she did not hold me, I could have easily collapsed. Matthew was on my right and, even though he is only eight years old, I could feel his support. At my back was the moral and psychological help of little Rachel. I could feel her little hands pushing me along and they felt so good. When I got home, I immediately laid down to rest. The pain in my back began to subside. In about two hours my resilience returned and before I knew it I was back again to me old cheerful self.

It has always amazed me how I am able to come back despite my pain and exhaustion. I call it my Lazarus self. I have tried to analyze it. I have tried to understand how I am able to recover, but I do not have a reason. For my entire life from the time I was a young boy, through my service years and my working career I have been able to come back with a determination and strength that even surprises me.

I know people my age with my afflictions would not take the chance of traveling around the world, but I have the ability to push myself and just keep on going.

7. A Traveler's Prayer to my wife:

My Heart will Go On and On

I think it very appropriate to complete this book with a special tribute to my partner, lover and pal who shares the trip with me. Here's the one I wish I wrote sung
by Celine Dion:

Every night in my dreams, I see you, I feel you
That is how I know you go on and on.
Far across the distance and spaces between us.
You have come to show you go on and on.

Near, Far, wherever you are,
I believe that the heart goes on and on.
Once more you open the door
And you are there in my heart,
And my heart will go on and on.

Love can touch us one time and last for a lifetime.
And never let go 'til we're gone
Near, Far, wherever you are
I believe that the heart goes on and on.
My heart is with your heart forever and ever.

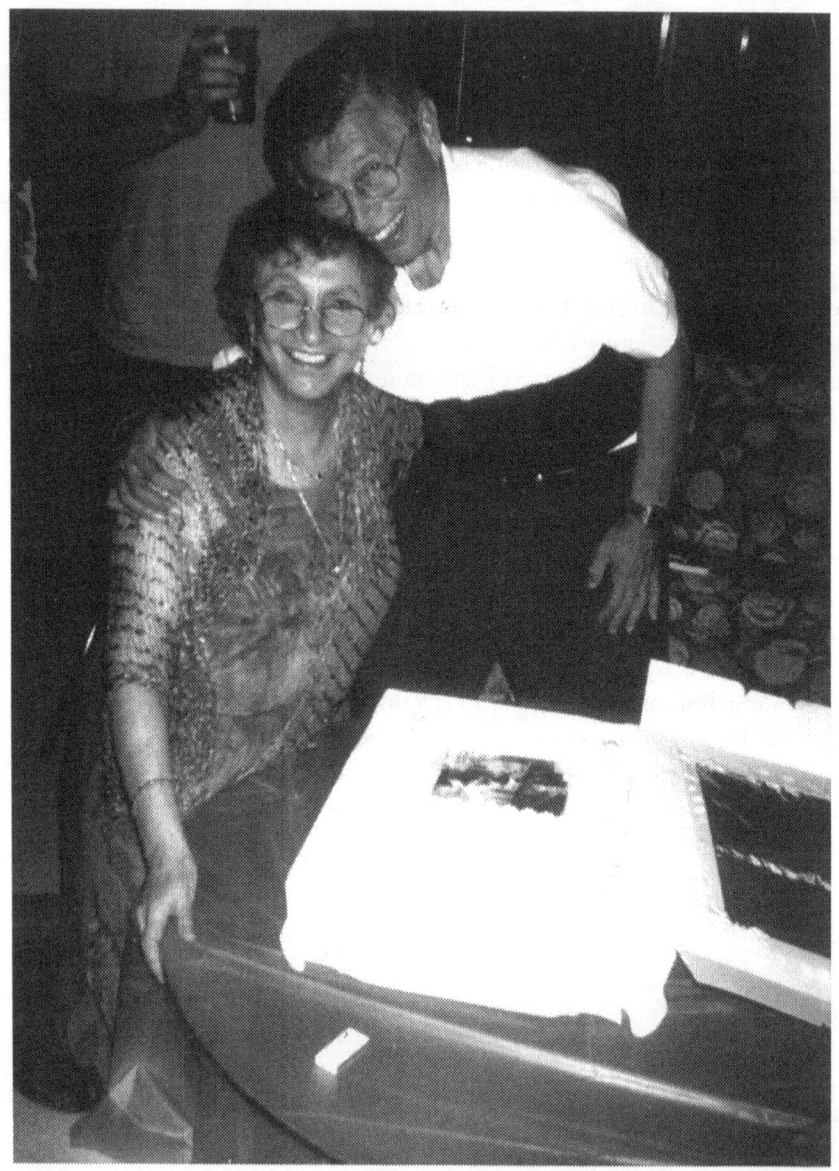

Gene and Lila at Chinese Walking Stick
Book Signing Party

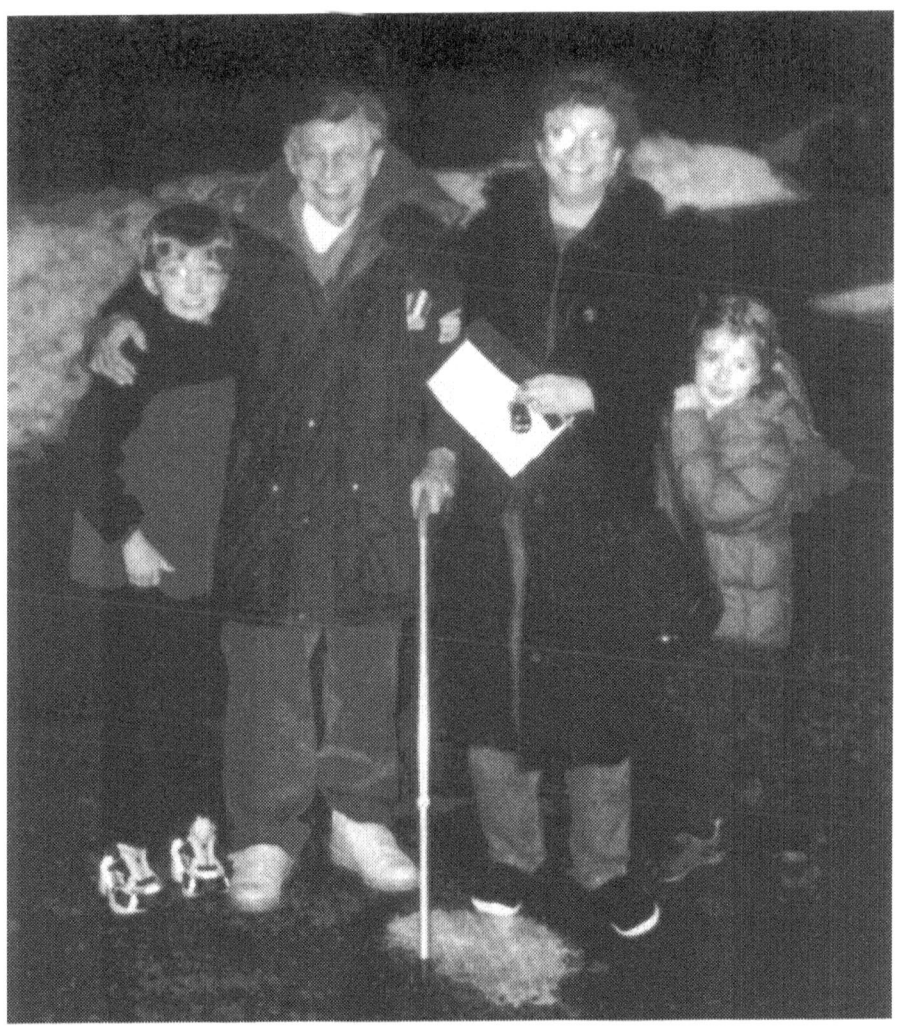

Going to 77th Birthday Party

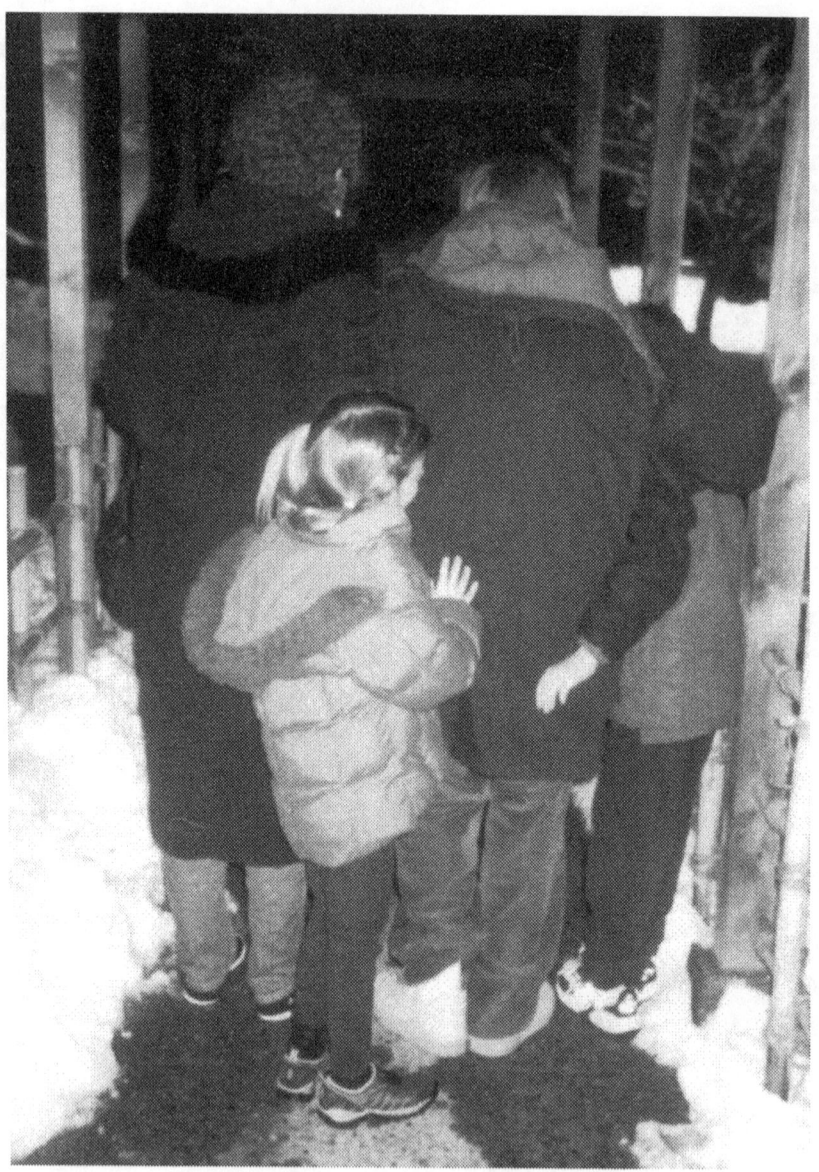

Leaving the Birthday Party

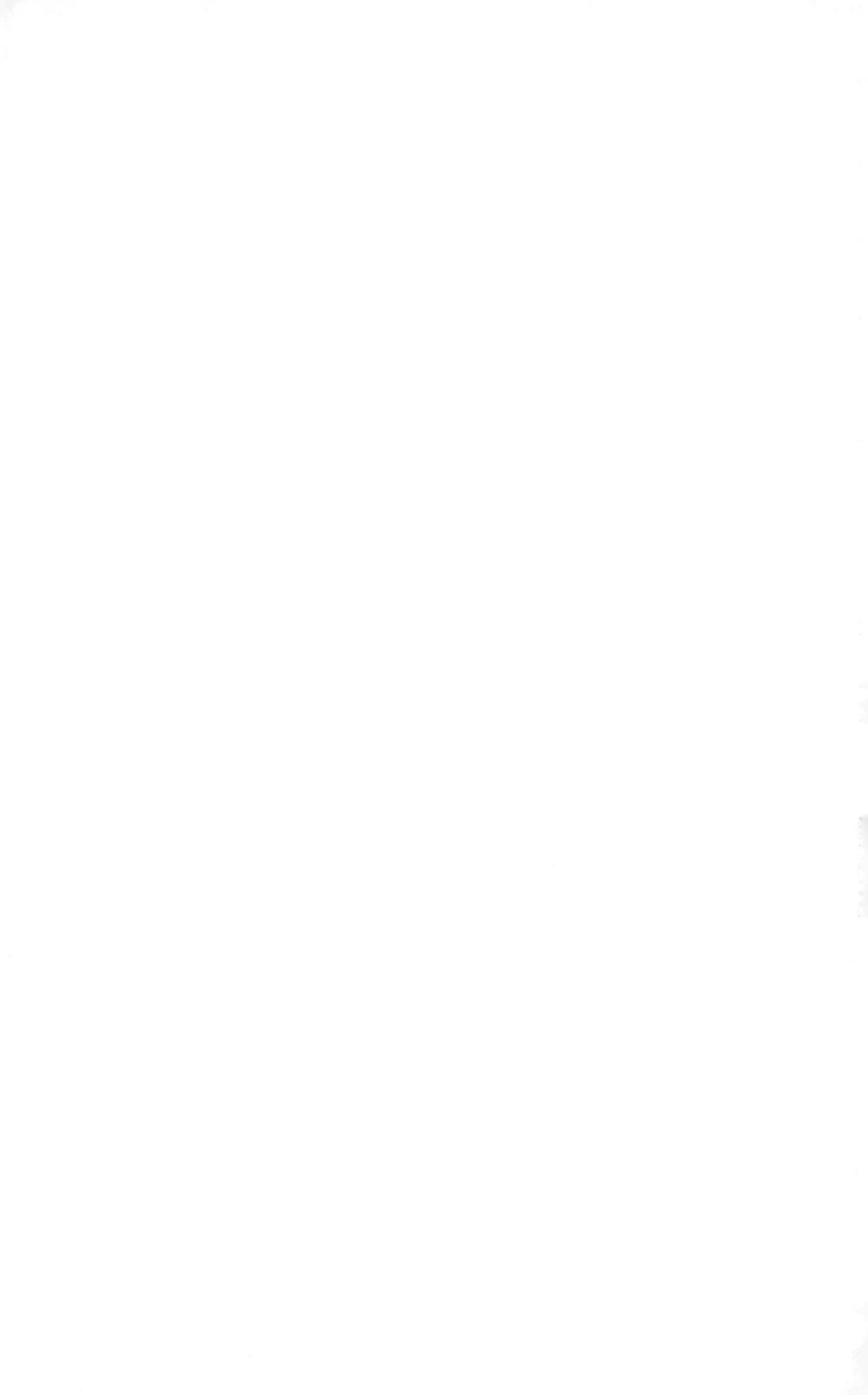

0-595-31560-7

www.ingramcontent.com/pod-product-compliance
Lightning Source LLC
Chambersburg PA
CBHW061257280526
45784CB00002B/800